Seeing the Unseen

A Past Life Revealed
Through Hypnotic Regression

Seeing the Unseen
A Past Life Revealed Through Hypnotic Regression

by
Ormond McGill

Crown House Publishing Limited
www.crownhouse.co.uk
www.crownhousepublishing.com

Crown House Publishing Limited
Crown Buildings
Bancyfelin, Carmarthen, Wales, UK, SA33 5ND
www.crownhouse.co.uk
and
Crown House Publishing Company LLC
P.O. Box 2223, Williston, VT. 05495-2223
www.crownhousepublishing.com

First published 1997. Reprinted 2007, 2008, 2010 and 2013.

British Library Cataloguing-in-Publication Data
A catalog entry for this book is available
from the British Library.

ISBN: 9781899836055

LCCN: 2003104686

Printed in the United States of America

Dedication

This book is dedicated to two lovely women, Katharine Bates (1857-1914) and Sarah Channing (1957- ???), who have lived in different times, different space, and different bodies. Yet they seem to be the same soul bringing almost forgotten subconscious remembrances into the world, offering insights showing a potential of new dimension of life beyond death in *Seeing the Unseen.*

Table of Contents

Acknowledgments

This book could not have existed without my wonderful client Sarah Channing who so elegantly recited her story of her previous lifetime as Katharine Bates. I also have to thank her for her permission to quote extensively from the sessions that I had with her and to reveal my confidential notes made during and after each session. And a great big hug and again many thanks Sarah for your co-operation without which the Postscript to this book would not have been possible.

I wish to thank all those who have been involved in the production of the book. These include Alexandra Harry and David Bowman at Anglo-American Books. A particular thanks to Jan Foxton for her work in editing my original transcripts and turning them into a neatly structured and readable document.

Again many thanks to Mark Williams for his brilliant work on producing such a stunning cover which so neatly sums up what my book is all about.

Many thanks to my good friend Dr. Martin Roberts for his Foreword and Postscript which add valuable additional colour both to the story and to the methods that I use.

Finally a great big hug to Glenys Roberts in Britain from both Sarah and myself for all the work she put in to researching the history of Katharine Bates. When this book was first written no one knew for sure if Katharine had ever existed on this earth or was just some figment of Sarah's imagination. Now we know that Katharine was real, all thanks to Glenys' tireless and painstaking research.

Preface

IS IT FACT OR FANTASY? This book is written directly from tape recordings made in my office. It consists of fifteen consecutive Hypnotic Previous Lifetime Regression Sessions recounting the experiences of a female subject's autobiography of a previous lifetime as another female personality seen on this planet for a time period from 1857 to 1914, while the subject was entranced in profound hypnosis.

For those of you who may want to take their research further and attempt to positively identify Katharine Bates or the people and places mentioned in this book, **Seeing The Unseen**, a few words of warning. A large proportion of the material in this book has been derived from audiotapes recorded during hypnotic sessions. Whilst the recording quality was excellent the client was talking in trance, mostly very coherently, occasionally quietly but always in a refined Oxford English accent. The accent alone gave me (a Californian born and raised) occasional problems in transcribing places and names absolutely accurately. I trust you will allow me a little licence in this respect.

I have included my method of handling PreLife Hypnotic Regressions in the text, along with my clinical notes.

Ormond McGill
Palo Alto, California
January,1997

Foreword

I count it a great honour to be invited by the author to provide a Foreword and a Postscript to this book. No doubt many will already know of Ormond's work as a therapist and as a stage performer, both with magic and with hypnosis, and a few readers will also be aware of his work in the fields of entomology and conchology. His achievements are truly legion, as are the accolades and endorsements which he has received for his work in all these areas and others over the years. However, his knowledge, skill and practice as a metaphysician perhaps exceed all of these.

Ormond several years ago became an octogenarian. However, when you meet and talk to him you find a person with the extremely active and agile mind more usually found in someone half his years. He still travels the world, passing on his knowledge to others through his workshops and seminars. He is a gentle man in the truest sense of the word, highly respected by his peers, adored by his students and much loved by those of us whom he has touched on our journey through life.

In the front of this book you will find listed some of the many books that Ormond has authored or co-authored over the years. This list is far from complete as there are many more works which are no longer in print and so are not listed here. Ormond first started to write this book in 1994 by transcribing the audiotapes of many hypnotic sessions he had had with a lady client. The client had been placed in a deep and profound state of hypnosis clinically known as somnambulism. It is in this state that subjects are most frequently observed to regress to earlier times in this life and, when appropriate, even further back into previous lifetimes. Such was the case with this particular client. Ormond was so deeply impressed by her story that he felt a permanent record should be made, which has now become this book.

Case studies have provided major contributions to nearly all schools of psychotherapy by demonstrating precisely what is occurring in a given situation. Often, however, the master practitioner does not provide us with his detailed case notes nor his innermost thoughts about his methods or precise details about the subject of his ministrations. In this case, in addition to recording all the content of the sessions, Ormond provides us with his full set of clinical notes which he recorded during or immediately after each session. He has also given us his preferred hypnotic induction methods used in all the sessions involved in this study. As a bonus he has also included another induction for those occasions when pastlife regression was his key objective. His method and his notes are, he feels, just as important as the story that unfolds.

Much has already been written on the subject of reincarnation, past lives and channelled messages. It is not for me to offer suggestions as to whether such happenings are real or imagined. I am content to leave such discussion to others who possess more knowledge than I in these areas. However, I am absolutely convinced that regression into a past life whilst in a state of trance can and often does provide an incredibly powerful healing agent for a great many people. For those seeking tangible evidence of past life regression, the bibliography at the back of this book provides a starting point for further research.

How and precisely what happens when a successful healing occurs through this medium is a matter of conjecture. Many theories have been put forward, but anyone attempting to provide a provable scientific basis to support their claims would almost certainly be on a fool's errand. However, one must also bear in mind that very little can be scientifically proven about the state which we call hypnosis. Much of the learned work in this field has been concerned with measuring brain-wave patterns during trance and attempting to describe the various levels or depths of hypnosis that are achievable. Considerable work has also been produced on the application of trance states, ranging from helping people with phobias or stopping smoking, through a wide spectrum including amputation and major surgery without the need for chemically induced anaesthesia. Unfortunately provable scientific evidence is lacking to support most of the theories which describe what actually occurs within clients whilst they are in trance. At best most of these theories or attempted explanations largely take the form of metaphor or allegory, whilst the unexplained proof remains hidden within the client who has benefited from hypnosis.

For nearly a century psychologists and psychotherapists have agreed that we are who we are and what we are largely due to the happenings and experiences that have influenced us since the time when we were born. There is no doubt that we also bring with us into this world other characteristics inherited through the genes donated by our parents. For those with a belief in past lives it is logical also to bring aspects of previous lives from the past into this life. However perhaps the real truth lies in the previous sentence within that all embracing metaphor itself contained within the word "belief".

A close parallel exists concerning double blind trials of drugs and the well-known and well documented conundrum which we have named the "placebo effect". In these trials patients are normally divided into two equal groups on a purely random basis (creating blind No. 1). One group is then given the drug to be assessed for its efficacy, and the other group given an identical looking pill (the placebo) which contains an inert substance with no drug content at all (blind No. 2). Always a number of patients who are given the placebo will respond positively to the dummy drug. In some trials over thirty percent have responded in this way.

We are still no nearer providing a wholly acceptable scientific explanation for this phenomenon than we were when it was first discovered. If we were, then perhaps the need to prescribe active drugs could be significantly reduced, with in many cases an inert placebo being prescribed instead. However, progress is being made, as it is now widely accepted that the placebo effect is a psycho-somatic phenomenon and not just a spontaneous physical reaction unconnected to the mind, as was widely believed only a decade or so ago.

Clearly what is happening in both these instances has to start at the psychological level (Rossi & Cheek, 1995). Perhaps the nearest we can get to a generally accepted explanation is to say that, at a level deep within our psyche and way out of conscious awareness, a shift has occurred involving our core beliefs. The consequence of this shift is that the process of self healing has kicked into gear or perhaps has become supercharged in some way that as yet we do not completely comprehend (Rossi and Rossi, 1996).

Having quoted from Rossi in 1996, and in order to place this in clearer perspective, I think it is pertinent to provide a quotation from Erickson & Rossi fifteen years earlier in 1981:

"Since ancient times, healers have been aware of the effects of words and ideas upon our physical well-being. Ideas can evoke real, dynamic physiological responses: hence the term *ideodynamic* to designate all the relation-ships between *ideas* and the *dynamic* physiological responses of the body. In the history of hypnosis, four stages have been recognised in the evolution of ideody-namic communication and healing:

Stage One: The medieval periods of prophecy, divination and magic.

Stage Two: The beginnings of hypnosis and the theories of the Chevreul pendulum and ideomotor movement in the 1800's.

Stage Three: Behaviorism and the clinical rediscovery of ideodynamic movement and signalling in the 1900's.

Stage Four: The psychobiology of ideodynamic healing in

hypnosis." (Erickson & Rossi 1981).

Perhaps then as we stand on the brink of the twenty-first century we are ready for Stage Five, a scientifically provable understanding of how our core beliefs and our presuppositions influence our bodily functions. Or perhaps we need to return to Stage One to rediscover learnings lost in the mists of time - learnings including those involving past lives. In either case, I am certain that eventually time itself will provide the answer to these and many other unsolved questions relating to hypnosis and trance states.

For the moment, however, enjoy this wonderful book for the knowledge that it provides about a method for uncovering past lives and the possibilities that this engenders. Whilst on your journey of discovery, do remember not to forget to enjoy the underlying and very interesting story from the nineteenth century.

Introduction

From one point of view this is a spooky book. From another point of view it is a spiritual book. In fact it is about spirits; indeed, the religion of spirits, SPIRITUALISM. Spiritualism had its heyday in America from the mid-19th century to the first ten or so years of the 20th century. Like every religion, much about it is subjective and requires aspects of faith to accept it. What is interesting is that the religion of spiritualism actually has more objective phenomena associated with it than do most other faiths.

During their heyday, spirit seances became a national social pastime. Even in the White House, seances were held. Mostly they were of a table tipping and rapping nature, in which a group of people would sit around a table (often a big one) and rest their hands upon its surface. The room would be darkened, and spirits would be asked to come and answer questions for the sitters.

Surprisingly often the table would commence to tip and move, and sometimes raps were heard. A communication was developed between the sitters and the table in which a "spirit code" was agreed upon: one rap or tipping to mean "yes" to a question; two raps or dips to mean "no"; and three "maybe" or "uncertain". The diversion was looked upon as a communication with the spirit world, and was lots of fun - a sort of mutual, social fun together that people enjoy, such as in the playing of a game of bridge.

Today we have television to amuse us, but in those early times seances were very much in vogue. However, don't for a moment get the idea that interest in spiritualism is entirely dead. It is surprisingly alive in the world of today. Thousands still adhere to the belief that we can communicate with loved ones who have passed on to the unseen world – often referred to as "the other side". Thousands very much believe in all manner of psychic happenings.

Just check in the *Yellow Pages* and you will find one or more spiritualistic church listed in every major city in the western world.

This book, **Seeing The Unseen**, tells about spirits and psychic phenomena in a very personal way. It is a book that will thrill and amaze you, arouse an angry spirit of contemptuous disbelief, and then compel you to admit that very possibly these things may be true. At all events, this autobiographic account of the lifetime of Katharine Bates brings in an eerie realization that we are living in a world of which we know little, but sense a lot. It brings in a conception that we actually have but a very limited glimmering of the real magic and mystery of life.

Seeing The Unseen, by its very personal nature and obvious honesty, may well effect a permanent breach in the high wall of self-protection with which many people have surrounded themselves, trying to keep out the unseen world: fearing lest they see, hear, and believe that Shakespeare was right when he wrote: *"There are more things in heaven and earth, Horatio, than you have ever dreamed of in your philosophy."*

What especially interests me about this book is that, while I wrote it, I am not its author. I will explain:

I am a hypnotherapist by profession, and pastlife regressions have become very popular with the public. Many people who believe in reincarnation want to be hypnotized to trace back subconscious memories which spring forth, telling of adventures in past lifetimes. Sometimes these recalled memories are pleasant and gratifying. At other times they can be disturbing and terrifying. But all are interesting. Some clients in my office articulate them very well, while others merely mumble. What are these deeply buried memories, really: are they fact or fantasy? Who can say? However, the fact is that they seem to help many clients to do a sort of mental "house cleaning" to pursue their life more clearly in the here and now.

My friend, clinical psychologist Dr. Edith Fiore, has been a pioneer in relation to this kind of hypnotherapeutic work, and has dealt with many cases of previous life regression. Her book, *You Have Been Here Before* [see Bibliography], tells of such in detail, and leads the way to sincere study of this important psychological field for research.

This story came through a client who was a somnambulist and went into a deep hypnotic trance. Her name was Sarah Channing (changed, of course, for her protection). She was an attractive young woman in her mid-thirties, and was exceptionally articulate in telling completely the story you are about to read. While in trance, she went back to a previous lifetime when she was known as Katharine Bates and - via session after session - presented this autobiography of her life, when she lived in the time of the heyday of spiritualism, and was herself mediumistic.

To me, as a person much interested in learning whether such subconscious experiences are based in fact or fantasy, what she has to tell while in profound hypnosis presents some of the most objective evidence I have yet to run across that indicates these past lifetime memories are based more in fact than fiction.

Before I present this case, exactly as it was recorded in detail as an autobiography, I will devote a chapter to explaining the past life regression method I used in this case, along with useful suggestions to assist other professionals interested in investigating and probing into this field of research.

Such will provide a scientific background to the detailed case related.

My PreLife Hypnotic Regression Method

Throughout my career as a hypnotherapist it has always been my practice to keep notes on each session I have with my clients. The process of gathering this information starts with my receptionist who asks each client to complete a short questionnaire, much of which just requires my client to tick relevant boxes. It mainly covers such areas as their personal details, brief medical history and other relevant information such as whether they ever been hypnotised before. Most clients can complete the form in around five minutes. I find this form-filling process serves several purposes:

a) It focuses my client's mind on the purpose of their visit.
b) It provides me with most of the basic information about my client which helps me to gain a rapid understanding of my client's background.
c) It relieves me of the task of having to write down a lot of detail, and leaves me free to totally concentrate on my client's needs.

Following the usual introductions and explanations about hypnotic regression I usually add a few notes to my client's file which I think are relevant. During this process I always carefully re-check to ensure that my client is a fit and proper subject for such an hypnotic exploration. This is important as the very process of induction can on very rare occasions produce adverse effects. I am particularly interested in identifying those subjects who are taking certain drugs (prescribed or otherwise) or who have a history of mental disorders and those who are prone to epileptic fits. If either my questionnaire or my follow-up questions reveal someone whom I feel would not benefit from hypnosis I decline to accept them in the gentlest possible manner and usually suggest an alternative therapy as being more appropriate.

When I am ready to start the session I ask my client to relax comfortably on a couch or recliner. The lights are lowered so the room takes on a twilight glow. Via a cassette recorder I play some relaxing music softly, as a background to the session. It is a soft, dreamy type of music of a meditative nature. The client is requested to close their eyes and just let their mind drift and go in any direction it wants to go. There is no attempt at control. Absolute freedom is allowed. I allow five minutes for the client to sink into this relaxed reverie state. I observe the client's breathing and, as it becomes regular and deepens, I begin the session with these personal instructions, spoken very softly directly into the ear of the client ...

"You are ready now to commence a journey and adventure back into your past. Begin by focusing your attention on your breathing ... breathing in white light ... feel it entering your nostrils ... going into the back chambers of your nose ... down your throat and trachea ... into your two lungs ... and inhale and exhale this white light.

"Feel your lungs expanding and contracting – inhaling and exhaling white light ... and, as you do this, notice that you're becoming more and more relaxed ... more relaxed with each breath you take ... each breath is a signal to your mind and body to relax ... to relax ... and, as you are relaxing deeper and deeper, in your mind's eye visualize yourself surrounded by a brilliant, dazzling, radiant white light ... and know that this light protects you in every way from any negativity or harm as you drift back into your subconscious memories ... and recall events in a lifetime you lived before.

"You are absolutely safe in the sanctuary and protection of the WHITE LIGHT. Sense yourself as encased in a warm cocoon of this protective white light.

"Now, use your imagination and feel the relaxation from your closed eyelids flowing down onto your temples like a warm, golden, relaxing liquid ... feel it flowing onto your cheeks, relaxing your cheeks ... down around your mouth,

onto your lips. Now direct your attention to relaxing your nostrils; see if you can detect that slight difference in temperature between the air that you inhale compared to the air that you exhale ... and now feel that warm, golden, relaxing liquid flowing over your temples again and feel it crossing your forehead, relaxing your entire forehead ... feel it flowing back throughout your scalp ... relaxing completely the muscles of your scalp ... feel it flowing down the back of your neck ... around the sides of your neck ... and the front of your neck. Feel those muscles just LETTING GO! Feel it flowing out to your shoulder muscles, permeating those muscle fibres ... feel it flowing down your arms very slowly, beginning with your upper arms ... your forearms ... wrists ... hands ... fingers ... and notice the tingling in your fingers. That's energy.

"Now feel that warm liquid flowing back up your arms and flowing down over your chest, relaxing the muscles under your skin and between your ribs ... feel it flowing down to your abdomen, relaxing your abdominal muscles ... down to your hips ... pelvic area ... genital area ... around to your back. Now, relax your buttocks ... now relax those long muscles on either side of your spine running the length of your back .... relax your spine by feeling that warm liquid flow through it, beginning with the base of your skull, flowing through each vertebra, relaxing the spinal nerves that come out of each one, all the way down to your tailbone ... and notice that your back is relaxing completely ... each muscle fibre j-u-s-t letting go ... and now feel that warm relaxing liquid flowing over your thighs, relaxing your thigh muscles ... over the calves of your legs, your ankles, heels, relaxing each toe – as you continue to drift down deep and deeper and deeper, totally relaxing ... totally letting GO! Going deeper and deeper than you have ever before ... just enjoying that feeling of increasing relaxation, peace and calm that pervades you. And as you continue to relax deeper and deeper, again use your creative imagination and put yourself in your favourite place in nature: perhaps it is next to the ocean ... in a field, on a mountain ... in a Japanese garden ... next to a brook ... now, look all around and see everything around you: notice the colors, the *shapes, the movement.   Notice something very near you. Now, notice something very far away.   Now look up in the sky.   See the clouds floating by.   See the birds flying.   Now, become aware of the sounds of nature surrounding you. Become aware of the scents and odors and fragrances. Become aware of everything that you can feel; perhaps you can feel the warmth of the sun smiling down on you. Perhaps you can feel a cool breeze blow across your face.*

"Now turn your attention to becoming aware of sensations in your body ... begin to feel your pulses beating in various parts of your body.   Now become aware of the taste in your mouth.   Perhaps you had a picnic ... something to eat and drink ... and feel yourself relaxing as you never relaxed before: total relaxation of your mind and body.   And now, again, use your creative imagination and imagine yourself going back through time and space, in a time machine, receiving crystal clear, vivid impressions from out of your subconscious memory banks ... recalling the things you want to recall ... the things that are important for you to recall ... things that are of interest and importance to your life in the HERE AND NOW.

"I am going to count from one to ten, and as I do, feel yourself going deeper and deeper as you go back through time and space with each count.   At the count of TEN, emerge from the time machine receiving crystal clear, vivid impressions.   Your inner mind is taking you back to the space and time to which you want, and it is important for you, to go.

"One, two, three;   back, back, back in time and space you go;   four, five, six;   back, back in time and space you go; seven, eight, nine, TEN: YOU ARE THERE."

You have now reached the place in your regression where you can use the images that come up for whatever the purpose of the session has been; possibly to just before the event or one of the events responsible for whatever it is you are seeking to correct.   Or possibly just to enjoy a pleasant recall of events of interest you experienced in a past lifetime. You can be absolutely safe in doing this reviewing of events, by assuring the client that such will be witnessed as in watching a motion picture or a television show. By using these instructions they will simply witness the event without getting caught up in it in any way.

This "witnessing" handling of the scenes that come up from subconscious memories is very important handling. Careless handling of bringing to recall (surfacing of) events in current lifetime and past lifetime has been a cause for concern for subjects reliving traumatic experiences from the past, and some law suits have occasionally resulted. All such traumas can be avoided by making the experience be one of witnessing and not getting caught up in reliving the experience. I always tell the client to remember that whatever is recalled is but a past memory, and that MEMORIES WILL NEVER HAPPEN AGAIN, WHILE THE FUTURE MAY NEVER HAPPEN AT ALL. AND THAT WHAT IS REAL IS THE HERE AND NOW!

If you will perform your hypnotic regressions sessions having the client surround themselves in THE WHITE LIGHT OF PROTECTION and knowing that they are entirely, simply a WITNESS to whatever comes forth, your regression sessions will be absolutely safe-guarded.

Having completed the session, and when ready to have the client return to the present time, suggest:

"Let go of these memories for now and return to the here and now. Your mind is bringing you back to today (give date including year). Again, use your creative imagination, coming back via your time machine as I count from ten to zero, coming back (person's name) ... to the here and now.

"Coming back to my office on this (repeat date) ... And as you come back go deeper still – with each count – so that I can give you wonderfully helpful suggestions which become the reality of your life. Come back today to the here and now:

"Ten ... nine ... eight ... seven ... six ... five ... four ... three ... two ... one ... ZERO! (Name), you are back today (date). Know that you did a beautiful job, that your regression was excellent and that you will remember everything you experienced today and more. And also know, deep within yourself, that each and every day, in every way, you are getting better and better. The entire quality of your life is advancing and improving in every way."

If working on the eradication of a specific symptom, you can add: the recall of the symptom you wish to make vanish in affecting client's life has been harmlessly brought up to a conscious level, and its subconscious influence has been removed from influencing client's life forever. Tell client that he (or she) is letting go of the difficulty forever ...that it is now being dealt with on a conscious level, rather than having it express itself unconsciously in a physical way. If you are not working on the removal of a specific symptom, go directly into this arousing technique

"Now at the count of three open your eyes completely and be totally alert and awake. When you open your eyes you will feel good all over and wonderfully alive, and you will KNOW THAT EVERYTHING IN THE UNIVERSE IS A MIRACLE AND THAT YOU ARE THE GREATEST MIRACLE OF ALL.

"Come up now ... you are back in the here and now (date) feeling wonderfully alive. IT IS GREAT TO BE ALIVE!

"ONE ... begin to move your body, stretch your arms and legs ... TWO ... take a deep breath ... THREE ... open your eyes completely now. You are totally alert and awake, back today (repeat date). What an interesting adventure in time this has been."

****

Such is the method of PastLife Regression I employ in my practice of hypnotherapy. Herewith is my CLINICAL HYPNOTHERAPEUTIC REPORT SHEET ON THIS CASE:

Client: Sarah Channing

Purpose of Sessions:
Fulfilling client's request to probe most pertinent events of previous lifetime of which she has occasionally had flashes of recall during dream sequences in this lifetime.

Hypnotic Responsiveness:
Deep somnambulistic subject. Responsive to posthypnosis testing with complete amnesia. Verbally articulate in describing recalled subconscious memories of a previous lifetime lived as another feminine personality – telling her story of living in that lifetime in a remarkably clear and detailed accounting of the time and space when she existed as Katharine Bates.

Report of Sessions:
These hypnotically induced prelife regression sessions, recovering past memories, were conducted approximately one per week over a period of fifteen weeks covering the client's life experiences as Katharine Bates from her birth (18 September 1837) to her death (28 August 1914).

****

Very honestly, I had no idea that what had started out as a casual probing of past lifetime dream sequences was going to develop into a complete autobiographic recording of her previous lifetime as the well-known historic personage of Katharine Bates, and so through a series of fifteen sessions (each session dealing with a different episode of her life) telling her life story from early womanhood to the conclusion of her life.

I have carefully preserved each recorded session, as her autobiography in that lifetime holds much of interest.

Having established that everything was in order with my client and also having checked to ensure that I fully understood what Sarah was expecting from me, I commenced the initial induction. Very rapidly Sarah entered a deep somnambulistic state of trance, closely following my every instruction to regress further and further back into the past as I counted from one to ten. On the count of ten Sarah took in an extra deep breath and then breathed out slowly whilst at the same time a smile spread across her face. This was a clear sign to me that Sarah had found what she had been seeking. I asked her quietly to tell me her name and was there anything she would like to share with me.

Here is my client's story when Sarah's soul dwelled in the body of Katharine ...

Chapter One:

ME, MYSELF AND I

Session 1.

I have always felt that I lived in two worlds: one seen and one unseen. The partition between the two, to me, seems paper thin. A physicist would call it a matter of vibration. This gift apparently is uncommon, and some have called me a natural medium. All I can say is that it has developed into a lifetime interest in investigating psychic phenomena and spiritualism, and has filled my life with occult experiences.

My name is Katharine Bates. I was born into a wealthy family in Oxford, England, in 1857 and died in America in 1914. Fifty-seven years was long enough for me to do what I needed to do in that lifetime. I gained something of an international reputation through my explorations and writings on the subject of spiritualism, which I have come to call our "unseen world". Some have called my writings somewhat brash but, honestly, I don't think I'm brash: rather I am the sort of person who likes to call a spade a spade. Along the way I have come to count among my friends such notables, in the "seen world", as Presidents Lincoln, Grant and Taft; Oliver Wendell Holmes; Sir Arthur Conan Doyle and other people the world acclaims, and, in the "unseen world", one famous friend stands out for me: George Eliot, whose spirit gave me the gift of SEEING THE UNSEEN.

My mother died when I was born, and my father (bless him), the Reverend John Ellison Bates, was both father and mother to me. We were devoted to each other. I suppose my interest in the unseen world was kindled when he died. I was nine years old at the time, and he had been an invalid all my short life. His last illness, which lasted scarcely a fortnight, came on suddenly, and he died quietly in his bed. His death came as no surprise to me, as I had dreamed for three consecutive nights that his spirit was soon to leave. In my dreams, I saw his inner self leave its worn out body behind on the bed. And when he died, somehow I felt him come close to me, and a warmth entered my heart in knowing he was very much all right. That was my first contact with the unseen world of which I was fully aware.

My nurse, elder brother and godmother were the only three people in my home at the time, and they gave strict orders that none of the servants should give me a hint of his approaching death. These instructions were carefully carried out. Yet I knew.

I will fill you in with a few details of my experience of my father's death.

How well I remember that cold, dreary February morning: England can be *so* cold and dreary at times in February. I remember being dressed by strange hands, and then my dear old nurse (who had been by his bedside all night) coming in and telling me the sad news, with tears running down her cheeks. As I have said, it came as no news to me, as I had dreamed for three nights that he was going to die. I had spoken to no one of my dreams for fear, I suppose, that they might come true if I did.

Perhaps there was some childish notion on my part that by being silent about my dreaming of his death I might avert the catastrophe. With all his previous illnesses I had never dreamed they would be fatal. In retrospect now, this was very likely my first recognition that I was psychic.

During the next few years of school life my psychic faculty remained dormant. In a fashionable school, surrounded by chattering companions, teachers and the usual routine of school work, there was little occasion for such perception. However, I do recall suddenly feeling that things around me were unreal, and that things just beyond my normal senses were the "real" reality. At such times I felt very alone in the world, and I found myself wondering if other children had similar experiences. I was too shy to ask: which was probably just as well.

I pass on now to the time when I was about eighteen years old and had my first formal introduction to spiritualism. I was a constant visitor in the house of my godfather, who was archdeacon of a northern diocese. His grandson, about my own age and then a young student at Oxford, introduced me to my first seance. His name was Morton Freer. It was with him that I sat at my first "table", more as a matter of amusement than anything else. Frankly, I must confess that we both treated the experience in a rather flippant manner. However, the table (I should say "spirit", as the table was just the instrument through which it manifested) did not seem to resent this, and some very interesting phenomena occurred.

In those days, I didn't trouble myself much about theories and, when we found that Morton and I alone could move a heavy, solid oak dining room table quite beyond our normal strength practically without exerting any physical effort at all, we looked upon it as an amusing experience without caring to enquire if the energy had been generated on this side of the veil or on the other side. All we knew was that we could move such a weight without exerting ourselves. We accepted the phenomenon at its face value without trying to explain the cause. Enough explanation for Morton and me was simply that "the spirits did it".

Now and then Morton's grandfather, the Archdeacon, would put his venerable head inside the room and shake it at us half in fun, yet with a good deal of earnestness, and I think he was more than doubtful as to whether our parlour games were quite lawful.

We were both very ignorant in those days on the subject of psychic laws. We performed what we performed in complete innocence, and probably that was our salvation; for I can remember no terrible or weird experiences, such as one sometimes reads about when inexperienced people try to contact the spirits. It was not until much later in life that I came to endorse most heartily the well-known dictum of Lawrence Oliphant – namely that, when he saw people sitting in an irresponsible way to "get messages through a table", it reminded him of an ignorant child going into a powder magazine with a lighted match in its hand.

Staying in the same house, I next recall a visit from my brother, on leave from India, who, while in America, had been introduced to important naval and military men and shown around the Washington Arsenal, West Point Academy and so forth. I remember well his look of amazement when Morton and I had lured him to "the table" one afternoon, and he was told correctly the names of two or three of these American gentlemen.

He was naturally sceptical and mentioned that he must have told me those names in one of his letters. I knew this was *not* the case, but it is difficult to prove a negative, so I left it at that.

Really it was a relief when my brother suggested what he considered a "real test", where any previous knowledge on my part would be eliminated.

"Spirits?" he said with a question mark in his voice: "Let them tell me the name of a bearer I had in India – he lived with me for some years – always returning to me when I came back from English furlough and yet, at the end of our close acquaintanceship, he suddenly disappeared, without rhyme or reason, and I have never heard from him since. *That* would be something like a test for your so-called spirits, but I know darned well they can't do it," he added cynically.

The three of us sat quietly around the table with our fingers resting lightly on its surface. Morton asked the question, and we waited patiently. Finally the table tipped at R, then at A.

"Quite wrong," my brother called out in triumph. "I knew it would be when any real testing came. *A* following *R* is definitely wrong."

"Never mind, Major Bates," said Morton Freer good naturedly. "Let's go on, and see what they mean to spell out." (Morton always referred to the spirits as "they".)

Fortunately we did so, with a most interesting result; for the right name did come through after all, but spelt in Hindu fashion and not the European way. That is, the name of this bearer was *Ram Din*, but Europeans spelt it Rham Deen, and my brother had entirely forgotten when the A was given that it had any connection with the man's name. When the whole word was spelt out by the tipping of the table, it came through completely as Ram Din. Then of course, he remembered, and then if ever there was a look of amazement on the face of anyone, it was on his face at that moment.

"Good God!" he exclaimed: "It is right on the button, and that is the real Hindu spelling too. I never thought of that when the *A* came at first."

(Speaking of buttons, I think this episode really knocked the buttons out of his scepticism for years to come!)

How did I explain it to myself? In later years, I have thought many times of this experience as a case that precludes conscious telepathy. Psychic investigators, such as Mr. Podmore, would be reduced to explaining that the Hindu spelling was latent in my brother's subconscious, though his normal consciousness repudiated it. I let it go at that.

Further inquiry of the table brought forth the information that Ram Din had died, was currently in the unseen world, and sent his deep appreciation of a longtime friendship.

Another curious incident – still more difficult to explain upon the thought transference theory – occurred in that same room:

One of the Archdeacon's nieces came to stay in the house about this time. She was considerably my senior and was very kind to me, with the thoughtfulness that an older woman can show to a sensitive young girl. This awakened an affection between us which has always remained. I recall our talking about the matter of marriage.

This was a time when marriage was looked upon not only as the most desirable, but as almost the only *possible*, career for a woman.

Her first name was Carrie so, when Morton, this lady and I were "sitting at the table" one evening, I said, with trembling eagerness, "Morton, ask if Carrie will ever be married."

I must mention that for some strange reason I fervently trusted that a Hungarian or Polish name might be given after the satisfactory "Yes" had been spelt out. But, alas, nothing of the kind occurred.

The table began with a *D*, and then successively *E, H, A, V* came through. No one ever heard of a Polish or Hungarian name of that kind, and I remember saying petulantly, "Oh give it up, Morton. It's all nonsense! Nobody ever heard of a *Mr. Dehav.*"

Once more Morton rescued a really good bit of objective evidence for the credibility of the phenomenon by his perseverance.

"Wait a bit! Let's see what's coming," he said.

By raps and tilts, letter by letter through the alphabet, the message came through. Admittedly a very slow way to communicate, but via the table was the only way we knew at this stage of our mediumship.

Frankly, I had pretty much lost interest in the experiment. Anyway, he went on to say:

"Let's see where this Mr. Dehav lives." He asked the question. This was answered by "Freshwater", and further information came through the table that he was a widower.

None of us knew any man who lived at Freshwater, so we regarded the experiment as a failure.

Several years later, however, my friend *did marry* a gentleman whose name was definitely Polish which began with the letters D E H A V, and he was a widower, and he *had been living* in his own house in Freshwater at the time we held the seance. She did not meet him until some years after our initial effort.

Mentally, I chalked up another "gold star" for the "spirits".

About the same time, but in the south of England, my attention was again drawn to psychic experiences by an event connected with the death of the famous Marquis of Hastings, of horse-racing fame. As a young girl, I lived close to the Mote Park at Maidstone, where his sister, the present Lady Romney, was then living as Lady Constance Marsham. The Reverend Dale Stewart and his wife (he was then Vicar of Maidstone, and I made my home with them for some time after leaving school) were friends of hers, and she occasionally came to visit them. On one of these occasions, when Lady Constance had just returned from paying her brother a visit, Mrs. Stewart remarked she was afraid the change had not done Lady Constance any good, as she did not look at all well. This was an unexpected remark to me, as I had always looked upon Lady Romney as an exceptionally strong and healthy woman.

She said rather impatiently, "The fact is that I did a very stupid thing the other day – something I have never done before – believe it or not, I fainted dead away for the first time in my life."

Asked for the reason for this, she explained that she, her husband, and Lord and Lady Hastings were dining quietly one evening together, "...When two guests, who were expected to arrive by train in time to join our dinner party, had failed to arrive.

"Looking up the timetable, our host, finding no other train that could bring them in until quite late, had the four of us sit down for dinner. While we were eating, we all heard a horse-drawn carriage driving up to the front of the house. We naturally all concluded it was the expected guests, very possibly coming in by another line.

"Lord Hastings said, "Tell our guests, who have just arrived, that we began dinner, thinking they could not arrive until much later, but we happily await them now to join us."

"The servant went to the door to invite them in. He flung open the door ready to deliver the greetings, but no one was there – no carriage, no horses, no guests. Yet, all of us had heard it driving up."

Lady Romney apparently took the event very seriously, remembering an old family legend, that when a horse-propelled carriage is heard to drive up – heard but is not there – it is an omen that someone at the head of the Hastings family is going to die. At the very thought, the impact was so strong that she fainted dead away, much to her embarrassment, as normally she is a very stable woman quite above superstitions.

Superstition. I have always considered myself above superstitions, so I let the incident pass. However, a few days later, while visiting friends in Buckinghamshire, I did mention it as a bit of humorous conversation. I laughed it off with, "Of course they had all been mistaken in imagining they heard carriage wheels and horses' hooves drawing up in front of the Hastings home." We all got a chuckle out of it, especially that Lady Romney had fainted.

To my bewilderment, three weeks later, all the newspapers were full of long obituary notices that the Marquis of Hastings had died.

A shake of the kaleidoscope, and I see another incident before me of direct personal concern:

At the time of the outbreak of the Afghan War, in the autumn of 1878, I was living with very old friends in Oxford. My brother, of the Ram Din incident, had returned to India and had been appointed Military Secretary at Lahore to Sir Robert Egerton, who was at that time Lieutenant Governor of the Punjab.

When the war broke out my brother, of course, went off to join his regiment for active service. However, I knew full well that there had not been time for him to have yet reached the centre of battle.

I was in excellent spirits about him, for he had been unharmed through many campaigns, and loved active service, as all good soldiers do. Moreover, I had just read a charming letter which Sir Robert Egerton had sent him on resigning his appointment as Military Secretary to take up more active duty for his country.

Yet it was just at this time, when there was literally no cause for me to have any special anxiety, that I woke up one morning with the gloomiest and most miserable forebodings about my brother. Nothing of the kind had ever occurred to me before like this, as he had been through many campaigns in India, China and Abyssinia.

My feeling was that a great and definite disaster had happened to him. I tried to throw the mood off. I told my friends about my intuitive feelings, and they told me to stop worrying about imaginary things.

But I could only repeat, "I *know* that something terrible has happened to him, wherever he is. It may not be death, but it is some terrible calamity."

I spent the day in tears and despair, and wrote to tell him of my feelings. A dispatch came back from the Military in India that my brother had been seriously wounded by a bullet entering his spine, and that he was helplessly paralysed. The date when he had been wounded was given.

Allowing for the difference in time between Quetta and Oxford, my mental telegram reached me in the same hour that my brother, while on a march some thirty miles beyond Quetta, had been suddenly struck down.

Perhaps now that I have studied more about psychic impressions, I could have received more complete details as to what occurred. However it could not have been more marked, nor more definite as regards the *fact* of the tragedy.

The time of his injury was in the early morning hours of 15 December 1878. The dispatch corroborating my feeling was in a letter written by a stranger in January 1879. Communication had been delayed not only by the war, but also by the fact that my poor brother was lying at the time deprived of both movement and speech, and could only spell out later, by alphabet, his message to his family at home.

....

CLINICAL REPORT

End of Session One. During the latter part of the session my client was clearly in a disturbed state whilst recounting the events concerning Major Bates' injury. Her telling of the events was interspersed with long pauses as though she was trying desperately to hear something, whilst at the same time her breathing became deeper and more pronounced. As soon as she had arrived at a point where her breathing had returned to normal I considered it appropriate to end the session.

I then gave my client a number of post-hypnotic suggestions to enable her to rapidly return to a deep somnambulistic state at the start of the next session. I also included a
number of suggestions designed to return her to the point
where she left off in this session. I do this for several
reasons but mainly to ensure that she returns to the same
past life rather than regressing to some other past life and
quite simply to save time in not having to carry out another
induction process.

She was then given the usual instructions to bring her out
of her reverie and back to the here and now. My client was
pleasantly aroused from hypnosis having no memory of
what she had said during this session, here presented
exactly as it was recorded in her telling. Subject was
obviously surprised at hearing the replaying of story of
these early episodes of her lifetime as Katharine Bates
which she had so lucidly recalled. Checked that she was
fully aroused and free from any latent tendency to return
to trance and ready to return to the world outside my
office. Presented my client with a copy of the audiotape of
the session, and the next session arranged.

Chapter Two:

MATERIALIZATION SEANCES
IN AMERICA

Pre-session Interview. I asked the client if she had replayed the tape of the last session and if she had anything she wished to comment on from the previous session or since. She said that she had played the tape several times and was very excited to have started her journey of exploration of her past. She also said that she had spent the last two days feeling very excited about this session and had felt a great desire to re-enter trance and continue to rediscover her life as Katharine.

Having asked her to relax on my couch and using the pre-arranged post-hypnotic signals that I had installed at the end of the previous session, the client relaxed completely and rapidly became somnambulistic. Once again she took a deep breath, exhaled slowly and smiled. A few moments later she recommenced the story of her life as Katharine Bates.

Session 2

It was in America that I attended my first professional spirit seance in 1885. It was a materialization seance – full materialization is beyond doubt one of the most striking of spiritualistic manifestations.

An interval of seven years occurs between the events I have thus far told about myself – in my lifetime as Katharine Bates – and my early psychic experiences. The years of 1885 - 86 were a fast-paced time full of wonder and excitement for me. Come along.

During those intervening years, nothing special of a psychic or spiritualistic nature occurred to me. Honestly, I didn't particularly wish any. The truth is that I rather looked back upon my early experiences of a mystical nature in the light of childish amusements more than anything else. Other interests had come into my life, especially in the fields of literature and music. Frankly I gave scarcely a thought to spiritualism.

During this time one little incident did occur in which I was introduced to a charming old man. He spoke of his dear friend, "Mrs. Jackson", whom he considered the only reliable medium he had met. He showed me some sheets full of hieroglyphics which meant next to nothing to me, although he said they were spirit messages from his dear departed wife.

It was all so much Greek to me (or should I say Egyptian!), and my only true sympathy for this elderly gentleman was with his obvious loneliness, and adoration for his wife's memory.

Another incident relating to a study of psychic things did occur while I was living with a Mrs. Lankester and her daughters in London. Her husband, Professor Ray Lankester, and his friend, Dr. Donkin, both had an interest in psychic things, and both were members of the British Society For Psychic Research. The talk of the day was the apparent exposure of the internationally famous medium, Slade, being declared a fraud in America.

When arranging my American tour, Mrs. Lankester kindly introduced me to a Mrs. Edna Hall, an old friend of hers who, while visiting in England, had been guest in their house several times during the period of the Slade trial. This lady was an American citizen with her home in Boston, and would you believe it, it was she who arranged for me to visit her native country, and persuaded me to attend a public seance being presented at the Civic Auditorium in Boston. She had been so helpful to me that

I naturally accepted the invitation. Before we attended, she introduced me to another of her Bostonian women friends, Mrs. Dorothea Porter. Mrs. Porter was an aggressive sort of woman who was a well-known figure in Boston society of the eighties. She was invited to join us in attending the public seance.

Well, to make a long story short, the three of us women went together to attend the public spirit materializing seance presented by the Berry Sisters (next to the Davenport Brothers, the Sisters were perhaps the most popular mediums putting on public demonstrations in the United States). Our hostess had pulled strings so we had choice seats, front row centre. Both Mrs. Hall and Mrs. Porter said they had no illusions about spiritualism, and considered it a fake. Mrs. Hall added that we would probably find it an amusing diversion showing the gullibility of human nature.

I make no comment.

As for myself, I approached the evening with an open mind. I tended to feel it would be a swindle. However I have never been a person not to acknowledge that there may be more things possible in heaven and earth than I knew in my limited philosophy. I knew that Shakespeare said something like that in one of his superb plays. As I kept a diary, I can tell you what occurred in general at the Berry Sisters' public seance.

The theatre was packed, and the auditorium buzzed with conversation. At 8.30 a gong was struck and the house lamps lowered. A hush fell over the audience as the stage curtains parted. In the centre of the stage stood a curtained cabinet.

The Berry Sisters duo entered together from the wings, and advanced to centre stage. They were tall slender women, each wearing a domino mask. One was blonde and one was brunette. We knew that the light woman was the medium and the dark woman the conductor of the seance. The two just stood silent for some moments looking out at the audience. Expectancy filled the theatre.

The brunette woman stepped forward and addressed the audience. She had a strident voice that rather grated on the nerves, yet did command attention. She began with the usual lecture telling of the cultivation of spiritualistic belief in America. Rather boring I thought, so I will move beyond it.

The front curtain of the cabinet was swished open, and the cloth hangings forming walls and rear were flung back, showing it to be just a framework of pipe. The entire structure was obviously empty. The curtains were replaced forming an enclosure. A chair was placed in the centre of the cabinet.

The blonde sister went inside and took a seat. She breathed deeply, closed her eyes and seemingly went into a trance. The front curtain to the cabinet was closed. Stage lamps were lowered so a twilight lighting filled the stage, with blonde entranced within the cabinet and brunette outside to conduct the show. Soft music came on to fill the theatre. The seance was ready to commence.

The cabinet curtains shook, and a rotund figure appeared as an ancient Egyptian priest. Well costumed. Very imposing. The figure was presented as the "spirit guide" for the seance. A man from the audience was invited on stage to talk to the guide. The man asked if the lady sitting with him might come up too. Permission was granted. Later, when I spoke to her, she said she felt a damp hand pass over hers.

From our group, Mrs. Porter was then invited up to speak to the priest. The Egyptian dashed behind the curtain and reappeared instantly as a younger man. He said he wanted to embrace her, and then decided that his love belonged to another woman in the audience – a striking redhead seated on the aisle. Mrs. Porter returned to her seat rather miffed, stating that he was not a good looking young man anyhow.

Mrs. Hall, Mrs. Porter and I kept careful eagle-eye watch as figure after figure came forth from the cabinet – each time to return into the cabinet, and when the curtain was opened only the Berry Sister playing the role of medium was seen inside, while the other Berry Sister was master of ceremonies. Mrs. Porter being the most aggressive of our group made several attempts to get back on stage to investigate, but she was invariably waved down by the master of ceremonies. She said quite firmly, "Will that lady in the front row please sit down. These spirits are not for her. Each spirit only wishes to communicate with its own friends, and she is disturbing the conditions, and is interfering with the smooth materializing and dematerializing of the spirits."

There were evidently numerous people in the large assembled audience who took the whole thing very seriously, as on every possible occasion they would call out, "Uncle Joe is that you ? How do you do, Gertrude?" and so forth. Were they sincere believers or were they paid stooges planted to excite the crowd? I didn't have the slightest idea.

One "spirit" appeared out of the cabinet as an old lady, dressed like a nun. She was introduced as Sister Margaret, who had taught English during her lifetime in St. Peter's School. A supposed student from the audience was invited on stage to talk to her, as a former pupil. She told of her spiritualistic experiences in such remarkably bad grammar, as to reflect small credit on Sister Margaret's teaching of the English language.

The girl said that Sister Margaret had appeared to her one night in a dream. She said her wish had been satisfied, and that she had been a firm believer in spiritualism ever since.

A young French girl, in draggy black garments and with a shock of thick black hair, then appeared out of the cabinet. She rushed among us in the audience trying to find someone to talk French with her. I spoke a little French, so I went forward and spoke to her. I took hold of her hands. They seemed to be ordinary flesh and blood.

The French girl spoke very rapidly, as if time were an object. She said she understood a little English, but could not speak it. Her mother had been French; her father, an Indian, *"un brave homme."* She returned to the cabinet, and was GONE!

As the materializing seance progressed, it seemed to me that a good deal of strange behavior was going on – embracing, kissing, that sort of thing. One old gentleman was constantly walking up to the cabinet to get embraced by a white figure, whose arms we could just see thrown around his neck, in the dim stage lighting.

The most exciting event of the evening, I would say, was when Mrs. Hall was called to come on stage: being told that a young man wished to speak to her. She became more and more indignant, and shouted it was a "gross imposture". The audience howled.

The master of ceremonies begged her to be patient and try to hear what the spirit had to say, but with a very emphatic "NO" she resumed her seat.

Finally we were told that three little girl spirits, whose mother was in the audience, wished to materialize and come through, but couldn't due to lack of children in the auditorium.

The mother seemed very anxious to see them, but suddenly the gas was turned up, and the seance was declared over – a very abrupt finale to a piece of unmitigated humbug, if I were to express an opinion.

I tell of this first adventure in America attending a public seance to show the sceptical frame of mind I was now in with regard to any investigation of spirit phenomena that might turn up. Also, the reaction of the ladies who had taken me to the seance only added to my own prejudice.

I subsequently became aware that the Berry Sisters had been exposed. There was merely a trapdoor in the stage beneath the cabinet through which the costumed people, as spirits, came and went. Not really very clever illusion work. However, in the light of my later experiences, very possibly my attitude should have been more hospitable to potential visitors from the Unseen World.

All of this gradually renewed my interest in a field I suppose I was really born for. I somehow began to long for the genuine spirit phenomena I had experienced as a very young woman. By nature I am a searcher. The next entry in my diary refers to a seance which I attended in New York a few days after my arrival there, and some two weeks following the Berry Sisters fiasco.

My stay in Boston had been longer than was originally planned, and I had the opportunity of being introduced to such outstanding people as Oliver Wendell Holmes, Colonel Wentworth Higginson and others of the Boston elite. Also my name had appeared several times in the Boston newspapers, as a writer from England.

Anyway, let's get back to the next seance I attended in America. Via the grapevine, I had heard of a certain medium in New York who was said to be very good. I was interested enough to go to New York to investigate. I went alone and found her to be a small woman, living in a small flat in an unfashionable neighbourhood. It was anything but impressive. Some eight people only were assembled in the extremely small room. All perfect strangers to me, but a fancied likeness in one lady present to a picture I had seen of Harriet Beecher Stowe led me to ask if it was she? I was informed my surmise was correct.

Most seances in America seem to favour the use of a curtained cabinet used to contain the medium, while the spirit manifestations occur within. In this small room there was no room for a cabinet, so a curtain was hung across a corner of the room to serve the purpose. We were invited inside to examine the alcove.

To commence the seance that night, the medium sat amongst us at first and said that a little child of hers, who had died some years back, was supposed to help bring about the materializations, but was never outside the curtains. She explained that if she came out herself, she might be able to help, otherwise she would have to remain inside the alcove. When in trance within the alcove, the young child's spirit could then assist her to assist others, and bring about visible spirit manifestations that all could see. I mention these things in the way in which they were told to me, offering no comment, but simply putting the case for the moment as spiritualists would put it. To do this, and then to give a faithful and unprejudiced account of what took place, seems to me the only fair way of treating such a subject.

I was told that too much concentration of thought on the part of the sitters was a deterrent to spirit manifestations. Possibly this accounts for music invariably accompanying such sittings. It seems to harmonize the circle, to relax all participating, and may also, unfortunately, serve to cover secret doings of dishonest mediums.

You see, my experiences with the Berry Sisters had made me suspicious, and I was on the lookout for trickery.

However, in this case, where the medium lived in a crowded flat on a second floor, there was hardly an oppor-tunity for the trapdoor theory. In a city like New York where flats abound, it would be pretty difficult to get downstairs tenants to put a hole in their ceiling!

As a matter of fact, there was something about this little woman that made me think that she was genuine. There was reverence there. Absolute silence prevailed when a spirit materialized.

I can corroborate the assertion that too much concentration of thought upon them proves a deterrent to the spirits for, on more than one occasion that evening, I heard a voice (quite distinct from the female medium) say gruffly, "Get the people's minds off us; we can do nothing while they are fixed on us so intensely." It occurred to me that *thought* in the unseen world corresponded to some *physical* obstacle in the seeing world of the earth plane.

This seance was getting interesting. It began by the medium seating herself within the alcove, going into a trance of some kind, after which the curtain was drawn across in front of her. An eerie glow appeared above the curtain, which was reflected on the ceiling of the room. Then the first spirit came forth (female), apparently the daughter of an old gentleman sitting near me. The form wavered a little and, for the old man, I was asked to step forward and help her materialize the "white veil", which all the spirits that came through that night wore. It was perfectly transparent, and I was told it is considered a necessary shield between the unseen world and earthly world vibrations - on the same principle, I suppose, that we put on dark glasses to protect our eyes from the blazing rays of the sun.

In my self-appointed role as psychic investigator and on the lookout for trickery, I thought that possibly the stuff – which was referred to as ectoplasm – might be a luminous gauze of some kind, which the medium had unrolled to produce the effect. But when I touched it, I knew differently. It was sticky and tacky, and little prickles went up my arms as I touched it. The spirit figure came fully out of the cabinet and stood before us. She held out her hands in front of her, turning them backward and forward that I might be satisfied that nothing was concealed in them. The soft, clinging material of her gown ended high up on the shoulders, so there were no sleeves to be reckoned with. I stood close over her, holding out my own dress, and she rubbed her hands to and fro over the cloth, and a sort of froth, like foam, lay upon the gown. It glowed for some moments, and then softly faded into nothingness. It was totally unlike any stuff I had ever seen in my life. The nearest I can describe it is like the very softest gossamer tulle that old ladies sometimes produce as having belonged to their grandmothers. But really it is quite beyond me to describe it accurately. I have no choice but to call it ectoplasm.

She was really quite beautiful, and finally took up the veil, unfolded it, covered her head with it and started to go behind the curtain. Just before she was gone, she turned her head to me and said, "Thank you".

Other spirits now appeared for the other people in the little room. Apparently all of these had materialized before, and they seemed to speak to various patrons there with comparative ease. One called "Angel Mother" (the mother of the medium) answered questions on spirit life in a loud American voice. Her answers showed a certain shrewdness, but there was nothing especially profound about them.

A male spirit called "Ned Seymour" (who in life seemingly had belonged to the Christy Minstrel Company) cracked jokes with a man in the audience, in a good natured but flippant and very unspiritual manner. Even various female spirits who appeared joined in with the undignified slang. It struck me that human beings are pretty much just as their development happens to be, on whichever side of the veil they are.

A little child came through and spoke in childish English, but used the expressions of a fully adult person. She described several spirits as "chying" (trying) to come through, but not being strong enough.

I was becoming sleepy, and was actually beginning to get tired of the performance (remarkable though it was) when my attention was once more roused by hearing that a very lovely female spirit, with a diamond star on her forehead, had appeared and asked for me; saying she had been a friend of mine on earth, and wished to communicate with me.

This was conveyed to me by the little child's voice, the spirit herself not having yet emerged from the curtain; but the medium's husband looked behind it, and told me of the diamond star, which he said was some "order" in spirit life in the unseen world surrounding us.

Having no idea who the friend might be, I begged for some further particulars before going up to speak to her.

"She passed from earth life about five years ago and in Germany," answered the medium's husband.

This was less vague, and now for the first time a suspicion of the spirit's identity crossed my mind; but I would not go up until a name had been given, and I asked for it before leaving my seat.

The voice of the little child from behind the curtain said that the spirit would give her name through her, and the process was an intriguing one. No one in that room other than myself knew the name I wanted given, of the girl friend I knew who had died in Germany. That was the proof I sought that these manifestations were real.

The little child voice began describing the name, describing it letter by letter, as you might describe the large capitals of a child's reading book. The first letter that came through I knew to be correct. The medium's husband asked if I was satisfied? I replied I would like to have the complete Christian name before giving an opinion.

In due time, the six letters of her name came through, spelling M U R I E L, and I had no further excuse for refusing to speak to the spirit.

I went up to the curtain, and she appeared in front of it. The man asked, "Would you have recognised her as your friend had no name been given?" To be perfectly honest, I found it difficult to answer that question, for the following reason: none of the "materializations" I saw had exactly a human face. There was no question of a mask or clever makeup, but if one can accept the idea of a body hastily put together and assumed for a time, the result is exactly what I perceived.

My friend in earth life was very pale, and had exquisitely chiselled features, and the ones I now looked upon were of the same *cast*. The height was also similar, and an indescribable atmosphere of refinement, purity and quiet dignity, for which she had been remarkable - all this was present with this materialization. More than this I cannot say, for no materialization I have ever seen could be truthfully considered *identical* with the human original.

I did not feel frightened, but I did feel embarrassed and naturally so, considering how unwilling my recognition of her individuality must have appeared. She seemed conscious of this, for almost immediately she mentioned her hands, holding them out for my inspection and saying:

"Don't you remember my hands?"

Now, as a matter of fact, my girl friend was noted for her beautiful hands, but she was too sensible to be conceited about them, and had too much good taste ever to make their beauty a subject of remark, even to an intimate friend.

I examined her hands, as she held them out to me. As evidence, although well shaped and with tapering fingers, they were as little identical with human hands as the face was identical with a human face.

Wanting to have something intimate to say to her, my first thought was for an only and dearly loved married sister of hers, also a friend of mine, and I mentioned in a guarded way, saying, "If you are really my friend have you no message *for your sister?*"

Without hesitation, she said, "Tell Jessie ...", going on with a message peculiarly appropriate to the facts of the case but of a much too private nature for publication.

Almost immediately afterwards, with no suggestion from me, she added:

"Poor Jessie! She suffered terribly when I passed onward so suddenly."

It struck me like a bolt of lightning that she had said "passed onward" and not "passed away". That is truth.

Her voice grew weaker. The spirit spoke feebly and with difficulty, "not having enough strength for more communication," she told me.

I moved in close and whispered to her asking whether her father (who had died a few months previously) was with her.

"Not yet," she said gently, "but I know that he has made the transition." She then kissed my hand, and faded away before my eyes; not returning to the curtain (close to which I stood), but vanishing into thin air.

The sitters in the little room were ecstatic. Everyone wanted to have a personal spirit come through for them. The seance was far from over, but I had had enough for my own satisfaction to know that the course of my real purpose in life was to learn, teach and tell all I could to those who were interested in knowing their true nature: that we are all divinely immortal in the reality of the seen and unseen realities in which we all exist.

This little lady, whose name I do not recall, was a medium towards whom I have felt a special warmth. Such a humble, quiet little woman was she, living in a very modest style, and yet there was a majestic quality about her that was transcendental.

I will pass on now to telling further of my adventures investigating spiritualism, during its heyday in America. Most assuredly I have never considered myself a professional psychic investigator, but I have always had a talent for it.

It was but natural that, while living in America, I should make some new friends. One such was an excitable Frenchman who, while somewhat interested in spiritualism, was very much filled with the same prejudice I had felt when I first arrived in Boston. I invited him to attend a seance with the little woman medium in the southside of New York. My thought was to overcome his scepticism. The results were disappointing. We went and sat together along with a few others but, while some phenomena did occur, it was not an inspiring evening.

My French friend, who had never seen anything of the kind before, came with an attitude of determined antagonism; this, plus his comparative ignorance of English and my feeble French, made explanations under the circumstances rather hopeless. The whole circle was put out of harmony, and a dead weight lay upon us all. Actually it was a relief to me when my excitable friend left, declaring that everything he had seen was *"physiquement impossible, mon ange"*.

He rose and departed so suddenly from the circle as to cause concern among the sitters that it might harm the medium. Everyone was agitated. However the medium remained quietly in trance, and seemed unperturbed.

Nonetheless, my French friend did serve a purpose in introducing me to Madame Schewitsch – a beautiful and charming Austrian woman – who, I am told, was of the Austrian aristocracy. Apart from this fact, which a mutual friend had told me, I knew nothing of her family history, nor whether she had brothers or sisters, dead or alive.

I had told her of my spiritualistic experiences with the excellent medium in New York. She was the kind of person who was not averse to believing in the *supernatural* but not before every possible *natural* explanation had been exhausted. At her home we talked some two hours regarding the pros and cons of spirit communication. Finally, she said laughingly, "Have you been to any seances lately?"

I said, "No," but that I would like to while I was still in New York. I rather wanted to get some "second opinion" outlook on the previous seance that had impressed me so much.

In a city the size of New York, every newspaper has a Personal column listing psychics, astrologers and mediums. I casually went down the list. A half-defined wish to see whether any spirit friend would come to me under different conditions and in a different part of the city, led me to copying out a spirit medium's address who offered seances nightly. Seeing this, I suggested we might attend one that night, but she declined. I was not too surprised as I didn't think she was very interested in this sort of thing. A couple of friends came by to pick me up and, after parting with the charming female Austrian, we went on our way.

While travelling towards home, I mentioned this medium, whose advertisement said she held seances nightly, and suggested, "How about tonight?" My friends said they were willing, so we turned about and headed for the medium's house.

The whole thing was unplanned. No one, including ourselves, knew we were going to attend a seance that evening. It was entirely the spontaneous impulse of the moment. This is important to remember as it adds significance to our psychic experiences.

The name of the medium we had decided to call upon was Mrs. Stoddard Gray. We arrived at her home and were ushered into an imposing parlour. There was a touch of elegance about the place. Mrs. Gray was quite a spontaneous medium. As soon as she entered to meet us, she looked at one of my friends and told her that there was an elderly lady standing near her but, of course, invisible to our eyes. Almost immediately Mrs. Gray began rubbing her knees, and complained of pain in them, adding "The impression of dropsy is being conveyed to me. This spirit seems to have suffered from a disease of that nature."

My friend took it all very calmly, and made no comment, but later, as we were driving to our homes, she said quietly, "It is curious that Mrs. Gray should describe an old lady standing beside me. My mother died of dropsy."

Other persons began arriving to attend the seance and, shortly after eight o'clock, the seance started. The assembled company in the parlour went into the seance room: it was a large room containing many chairs and in the front was the curtained spirit cabinet, which I had come to associate with spiritualism seances in America.

The lamps in the room were lowered; soft music came on; Mrs. Gray entered the cabinet and seemed to drop into a trance; a servant closed the curtain of the cabinet in front of her. We all solemnly waited for something to happen.

The first manifestation to occur that evening was the arrival of a "spirit", who came out from behind the cabinet's curtain to stand in front of it. The figure was dressed in a flowing gown which shimmered in the dim light. The servant pulled the curtain open and Mrs. Gray was there sitting still in trance. Gradually she came out of it, and smiled at us. The "spirit figure" still stood there.

"Does anyone in this room speak German?" the medium asked. "This spirit does not seem to understand English or French. German is her language."

I had taken a course in German while in school, so I volunteered to talk to her. The moment I went up to the figure she seemed to gain strength, and said to me in the most refined German (anyone who has studied the language knows there is as wide a difference between the highest and lowest type of German accent as between an educated Irish accent and an Irish brogue):

"Ich bin die Schwester von Madame Schewitsch," mentioning the name of the foreign friend with whom I had been spending that afternoon: *"Ich weiss das Sie heute Nachmittag bei meiner Schwester waren,"* (the translation of which is, "I am the sister of Madame Schewitsch – I know you spent the afternoon with my sister").

She evidently had an almost overwhelming desire to make some communication to me for her sister, but the difficulty in doing so seemed equally strong. I looked to where Mrs. Gray had been standing. That lady had returned to her seat within the cabinet, and seemed deeply entranced again.

Despite the lack of strength of the shimmering spirit, she spoke sufficiently audibly that I could understand perfectly her well chosen and well pronounced words in German. But some obstacle seemed to prevent her telling me what she really wished to convey, and the despairing attempt to surmount this was painful in the extreme.

I responded, and went forward to the "spirit" directly and very gently. I assured her of my willingness to help in any way possible, but all in vain.

"Is it that you are not happy?" I asked.

"No - no! That is not it."

It came to me that she was trying to convey some sort of warning that had some connection with illness, for the words *Achtung* and *Krankheit* (warning and illness) were repeated more than once, but no definite message came.

I asked if she could write it, and she responded eagerly to the idea. So I borrowed a pencil and some paper, and placed them on a small table in the middle of the room, with a chair in front of the table. Still glowing she sat down quite close to the table (five gas burners were half turned on, so there was plenty of light), took up the pencil, but almost immediately threw it down saying in a most unhappy and despairing voice, *"Nein! Nein! Ich kann es selbst nicht schreiben!"* ("No! No! I can't write it myself!") Rising she went into the cabinet and stood beside the medium. The servant pulled the curtain shut. That was the last we saw of her.

My experience with the Berry Sisters had made me suspicious so I thought possibly this might be some sort of theatrical performance, but then no one other than myself and my friends who had come with me knew of my visit with the Austrian lady that afternoon.

I reflected that, had this been a fraud, and supposing that somehow my visit had become known – by hook or by crook – what could have been easier than to give some commonplace message in a language of which she had already proved herself mistress. Just before the spirit departed, I heard a whispered, "I was a nun in earth life."

The episode was so painful that I decided not to write to Madame Schewitsch about it. I have therefore no absolute corroboration of the fact that the lady mentioned had a sister who had become a nun, and had died. However such is more probable than not, because in every highborn Catholic family in Austria one member almost invariably takes the sacred vows. There is a sequel to this episode which came to me while I was travelling in California. I received a letter from my sceptical French friend that Madame Schewitsch had suffered a serious illness, and had almost died. Fortunately she recovered.

To return to Mrs. Gray's seance.

About twenty minutes after the "sister" had disappeared, a figure in white came out of the cabinet and pointed towards me, saying quickly, "For you."

I went up at once, recognizing who it was, but determined to give no sign of this fact.

The "spirit" looked at me for a moment, in a most quizzical way, as one might look at any well known friend who passes them in the street without recognition, and whispered, "Surely you remember me. *I am Muriel.* I came through and we spoke together at a seance held in Southside New York, but a little while ago."

She made me feel ashamed that I had tried to play the role of sceptic, for of course I knew her – I had recognized her the moment she appeared.

I grasped her hands in mine (they had the same "there" but yet not fully "there" feeling that I had noted on her previous visit), and said with sincerity in my heart, "I am so glad that you have come through to me again."

She kissed me. There was nothing the least repulsive in the touch, although it was not exactly like a kiss given by anyone on earth, but had an indescribable atmosphere of freshness and purity, such as had always seemed to surround this friend while she had been alive and was still very apparent even under these changed conditions. Another little point is that I had entirely forgotten my friend's love of violets (she always wore them when possible, and used violet perfume), and I smelt them distinctly while speaking to her in spirit.

As I pointed out before, it must be remembered that until the day of the seance, we had never dreamed of going to Mrs. Gray's house, nor had we even heard her name. I picked it out of a newspaper advertisement column by chance – amongst at least thirty others.

Until around seven o'clock that evening we had not decided to visit her, and the seance began around eight p.m., no single person in that room in upper New York having been with me when I attended the seance on the Southside some weeks previously. Under the circumstances it would be difficult to account for the fact of my friend appearing again in spirit on the grounds of collusion between the two mediums. Moreover, such collusion would not account for the appearance earlier in the evening of the spirit claiming to be the sister of Madame Schewitsch.

No one of my acquaintance has been able to offer any intelligent explanation for my personal experiences on these occasions. Conjuring tricks, trapdoors and all manner of deceptive ideas are trotted out by the sceptic; but at least to me, who lived them, the experiences were genuinely spiritual.

As I am now chiefly concerned with giving an overall picture of various incidents in my life, I resist the temptation to go further into the phenomenon of *Materialization,* either from the historical or ethical point of view, and pass on to the subject of clairvoyance.

....

CLINICAL REPORT

End of Session Two. Used the same procedure as at the end of session one to reinstall post-hypnotic suggestions. However, this time being aware of her impatience to explore further, I also gave her some suggestions that she should do so only in my office. I did this not out of a desire to restrict her or for my own benefit but to protect her from rushing rashly into something that she might not be able to have full control over. Later there will be an opportunity to teach her how to explore safely on her own but not for a little while yet.

Client pleasantly aroused from hypnosis, having no memory of what she had said during this second session, when she was regressed back in time to her lifetime as Katharine Bates, telling of her first seance experiences in America. I have written of them exactly as they were taped in my office.

This was a very interesting session for many different reasons but chiefly because Katharine had many learning experiences during this period of her life as told by Sarah. It is possible that the learnings of Katharine could have a direct relationship to some psychological needs of Sarah. Sometimes past life experiences can be metaphorical in nature as though to give substance, reason or cause for some belief or behavior of the client in this life. Must check for this before the start of the next session. Session Three arranged.

Chapter Three

SEARCHING FOR CLAIRVOYANCE

Pre-session Interview. Asked client about her experiences since her previous session. She said she had played the tape a number of times and "was absolutely fascinated by what she had heard". Asked client if she saw any relationship between the life of Katharine and her own. She mentioned having a dream in which she had met Katharine in this life-time on a film set. She said that she didn't attach any meaning to this and just took it to be her mind trying to put things in some form of order. To allay any hidden fears that she might have I confirmed that this was probably the case. This could be a sign that my client is beginning to resolve a current or past problem in this life or it may have no meaning at all. Nevertheless I shall be on my guard. Client very keen to get on with the session so we did not delay any further.

Almost as soon as she was fully reclined on the couch and before I could turn on my tape machine she drifted into trance. In order to ensure that she return to her story as Katharine Bates I repeated the post-hypnotic signals that I had originally set up at the first session. A few moments later she recommenced recounting her life as Katharine Bates.

Session 3

My experiences with materializations provided excellent opportunity for observing the physical phenomena of spiritualism. My search in this period of my life was for the mental phenomena.

It was while I was touring the USA in the Summer of 1886 that I first seriously turned my attention to investigating the mental aspects of psychic phenomena.

Clairvoyance was my goal. Clairvoyance meaning, in defin-
ition, "clear seeing". My investigations have led me to
believe that this faculty of inner sight can best be used by
persons whose lives have been eventful, and less effectively
by those whose lives have been mundane. In my own case,
I seem to be an "open book" to clairvoyant perception,
which I suppose could be regarded as flattering. Personally
I have had numerous "readings" – some good, some bad –
but happily most have been truthful, beautiful and
descriptive of me. It has caused me to learn all I could of
this psychic art, related to the spiritualistic path I was on.

I will tell of a few personal cases, which I can report
accurately, as they are taken directly from my diary.

That there is a good deal of guesswork in clairvoyant
readings done even under the supposed influence of
"trance" is quite evident to me. I am not prepared to say
that such trances were not genuine, but the remarks made
during them were frequently of such a vague and general-
ized nature, that anything containing accurate and specific
detail was hailed with a huge "Hooray!"

On the other hand, many clairvoyant readings that I
have had have been splendid. As an example, I have been
told numerous times that my mother (who died when I was
born) was my guardian spirit, and six times her name was
given me: with some difficulty in one or two cases, but
invariably without the smallest guessing on the part of the
clairvoyant, or any hint from me.

One of my most successful readings was in New York
with a Mrs. Parks of Philadelphia – a very pleasant healthy
woman quite unlike the usual cadaverous, gypsy type one
tends to think of as being a fortune-teller.

Mrs. Parks' fee was rather high, and I complained a bit.
She simply said, brightly, "Well, don't come if you don't feel
like paying that, but I never alter my price. You will find
that I am worth it." I liked her confidence in herself, so I

paid the fee and was glad I did. She gave me an excellent clairvoyant reading. I will fill you in on some details:

After referring to my mother's presence as my guide, and giving her name without the slightest hesitation, she gave me several messages with regard to character which were singularly appropriate, and finished up by saying, "Your mother does not wish you to go too often to mediums or mix yourself overly with such persons. It is not necessary for you to do so. She says you have enough mediumistic talent of your own for her to be able to communicate with you directly."

I could not help saying, "Mrs. Parks, you are going against your own interests in telling me this message. I am a stranger in your city, and your reading for me has been so excellent I had planned to come several times more."

She laughed and answered, "That is quite true, but I am an honest woman, and I am bound to give you the message that is given to me for you. You see, I look upon myself as a mental medium, and what comes through me is of spirit."

I asked her how she felt about her work. She replied frankly, "I do what I do because I am summoned by forces from beyond myself. Ever since I was a little girl, I have known 'spirit voices' speaking to me, and telling things that I had no other way of knowing. It is a true gift, I know, but it does have its complications. My husband has always objected to it. He was afraid it might injure my health, and for two years I gave it up entirely.

"But," she added, "the spirits would not leave me alone. It seemed as if I *had* to come back to it, as if I were refusing to use what God had given me to help others. But I try to limit my work, which is why I charge a higher fee for my services than other clairvoyants do. Also, I shy away from persons who come just out of curiosity, and sometimes I am guided to refuse admittance to some persons entirely. As you are yourself mediumistic, I can tell you something I have told few others. Not only do spirit voices come to me in auditory form, but my eyes are equally perceptive, and frequently the spirits about are clearly visible to me. I know, as you know, it is possible to see the unseen."

I knew that Mrs. Parks was a wise woman, and that she told the truth. My intuitive sense told me so. Indeed, *I am* somewhat clairvoyant myself.

I must mention one or two more incidents connected with this period of my psychic investigations in America, because they throw light on some obscure problems.

While consulting these clairvoyants, in widely different parts of America, two very near relatives of mine who had passed onward, were almost invariably described: and the names – one male and one female – were generally given. The mediums invariably went on to say that the female spirit was more developed than the male spirit. Now this was completely opposite from what I personally had thought about the two people. To me, the woman's nature had seemed far more worldly, as it were, while the man's nature had seemed of high spirituality while on earth.

In spite of my conceptions of these two people, clairvoyants continued to make this "mistake" (as I honestly thought it was) in describing the nature of this man and woman. It certainly seemed strange after giving accurate descriptions of the two relatives referred to – names included – that each clairvoyant would insist that the woman was more highly evolved in spirit than was the man.

Some months later, in the course of my travels, I found myself in Denver, Colorado. I stayed there only a day or two to break my journey further into the Rocky Mountains. The previous day, when wandering about Colorado Springs, I came by chance (?) across a woman doctor and, having asked some trivial questions, revealed we had a common interest in psychic matters and was invited to her home, where we passed some pleasant time discussing such things, including spiritualism. I gave no account of my personal experiences, merely mentioning that I had some interest in the investigation of this subject.

Hearing this, and knowing I was due to return to Denver, this lady gave me the address of a young married friend who lived in that city and who had, during the previous two years, suddenly developed strong mediumistic power, but was in no way a professional. She begged me to call on her friend if possible, so I took down her address, but said it was doubtful whether I would have time to visit, in the short time there which I had at my disposal.

At the end of a long afternoon's sight-seeing tour, I found myself in an area of Denver not far from the home of my new friend's friend, so I called at the house of the young woman. The person who answered the door said she was sorry, but it would not be possible for her to come out to see me as she was delicate, and her husband seldom allowed her to go out at night.

As I was leaving Denver early next morning this made a meeting impossible, so I left my card, and a note to explain my visit. Then I returned to my hotel.

Going into the hotel office after dinner that evening, I heard a gentleman inquiring for me by name, saying he had brought his wife to see me. I explained that I was the person he asked for, and he went on to say, with rather stoical resignation, "I do not like her going out, but she insisted. So she is here to see you."

The lady in question came into my hotel room upstairs after dismissing her husband, and said that she "preferred a room already permeated by my energy". She then continued very simply, "I do not know whether I shall be able to help you at all, but it seems there is something you need to have explained. When I read your note I felt bound to come, although my husband tried to dissuade me. An important message from the other side that has confused you needs to be explained. It was as though spirits whispered that into my ear."

She went into trance and gave me a good "reading", ending by describing my relatives well, and making the usual "mistake" in relation to their relative spiritual positions.

This was all said in trance. When she came back to full awakeness I said, "Now Mrs. Brown (her real name), I must tell you honestly that you have made one cardinal mistake, but I confess that five or six professional mediums have done just the same, in looking upon the woman in the case as being more highly developed than was the man when just the opposite is clearly the case." I then asked if she could account for such a persistent misconception.

"Wait a moment," she answered, "perhaps the spirits will tell me."

She looked into space with an intent expression for some moments, then closed her eyes and began to speak in a sonorous voice, as though repeating a verbal message which was flowing into her:

"It has nothing to do with your earthly ideas of goodness. Spiritual life can only come to those prepared for it, within the limits of their capacity. The male spirit you ask about was a sanctimonious man, and a regular churchgoer, but he was *creed* bound. He has clung to his creed even here on this side of the veil. In this he is not a free soul, although his perception is slowly advancing, it is a happiness to say. Now his wife is an entirely different matter; she is a free soul who can play in the playground of existence. She is of a directly *apprehending* nature. She can see the light of truth more clearly than can he. She is on a higher plane. That is why you have been told so many times that she is actually more highly spiritually developed than is he. But she loves him and she will help her husband very much, and in time he will join her, and they will progress together."

Her explanation was given to me in a quick, decisive way. Now I understood. Never again will I judge an individual by outside appearance, when it is what is *inside* of each that tells of their true nature.

Later, in San Francisco, a clairvoyant referred to my friend "Muriel" – her spirit had come to me during two separate seances, as I have related to you. This medium described her in rather vague terms. When I pointed this out he said a little impatiently, as though we were wasting time quibbling, *"Oh well, it does not matter. The spirit tells me you know perfectly well who it is! She has already appeared to you twice in New York."*

I took two young friends with me to see this particular male medium. They were very sceptical and in a rather flippant state of mind. He described "the spirit" of an uncle who had come across for them, and gave further information that he was surrounded by water and was drowned; also that he was very musical.

This was received with laughter by the two young people; they declared it "balderdash" without a grain of truth in fact.

The medium looked mortified. I know he was glad when we left.

On our return home, when the young people were telling their mother the "balderdash" as they laughed, the mother said quietly, "Do you not recall, dear children, of my telling you years back of your Uncle Robert, who was drowned and died before any of you were born. He was a fine musician. He wanted to devote his life to music, but was persuaded to take up another profession."

I tell you of this incident to express the carelessness with which we sometimes can be determined to find fraud, sometimes at the expense of finding truth.

Before I close this accounting of my clairvoyant mediumship investigation in America during the years 1885 and 1886, I will tell you of one more personal experience.

While pursuing my psychic investigations in eastern USA in March and April of 1886, I was told there was a band of six guardian spirits forming around me, and that shortly these would be supplemented by another band of six further spirit protectors. Mostly one hears of such things as "Guardian Angels". Whether or not this has any bearing on the following adventure I honestly cannot say. Anyway, it went like this:

My search continued, and some three months after the time I was told of my Guardian Angels, I found myself on Vancouver Island, living for the moment in Victoria. I was not alone, for a girl of about my age, Miss Eleanor Greenleaf, had joined me as a travelling companion. She was an attractive girl with plenty of money and time to travel. Likewise she had an interest in spiritualism, having attended a number of seances.

As we lay on our beds in our hotel room quite suddenly I realized that I saw something strange in the air – just above and in front of my head. I mentioned this with such surprise to Eleanor that she suggested I must have eaten some indigestible food at dinner and was seeing things. At first I was inclined to agree with her, but shortly my opinion was altered by the fact that what I saw as an indistinct blur began to take on a definite shape. The shape I saw forming in front of me was of six little swallows, apparently connected with each other by a waving ribbon.

It was quite distinct to me, and I tested it by opening and shutting one eye at a time, which did not affect my vision. There they remained, both at that moment and for several succeeding years. Whenever I directed my attention vacantly into space they were there. I got so used to the habit of seeing them, I nicknamed them "my birds".

About six months after their first appearance in the clear, pure atmosphere of western Canada, I saw my six birds as usual, but the vision had increased, and where there had been six before, now another ring of six had joined them.

A few days later, in my vision, the new birds and the old ones had joined ranks, and now twelve little swallows floated in the air before my eyes. It needed the background of a clear sky to make them readily seen. I know it sounds rather strange but, as they provided comfort to me, I just accepted them for whatever they were. I guessed they were my promised protectors that I was seeing through my developing clairvoyant powers. One doesn't mind having visions of "protectors", so I let it go at that.

In my study of clairvoyance, it seems that frequently such psychic impressions come in the form of symbols.

Subsequently other visions have come in. One was an anchor with a chain attached, and on one end of the chain was a short hook. Near the anchor I sometimes saw a sacrificial altar with flames rising up; then a triangle with loops at the corners, which I was told was the sign of Nostradamus. Another was a vision of an old mirror in a quaintly shaped frame, and finally there was a vision of a long staff, with the sign of Aries at one end. I have since realized that this is much like the "Staff of Faith" found on the tops of many tombs in the Roman catacombs. All of these visionary emblems somehow seem to be connected by a ribbon binding them together. I cannot see them at will, but when the atmosphere is right they come in bright and clear.

What are these clairvoyant visions? All I can say is that I find them comforting, and it is fun to try to guess their meaning. One clairvoyant also said they have connections with my past lives.

Denver was my next stop, where Eleanor and I were separated after a year of being together. She was going back to San Francisco to take a steamer for New Zealand, and then go on to Australia. My plans were to return to England for family reasons.

After she left, I came to realize how much her friendship had meant to me. I would have felt far less lonely had my journey East corresponded more closely with her journey West.

Waking early and lying in bed, feeling very melancholy at the idea of being left behind and alone in the very centre of America, I looked up and, to my delight, saw a new sign. Not little birds this time, but two big father and mother birds, with a short string attached, not horizontally as before, but perpendicularly. At the end of this short string was a tiny bird, even smaller than the swallows, evidently being guided by the two big birds and quite safe in their charge.

I found a pencil and made a rough sketch of the vision. This was fortunate or I might well have imagined that I had never seen it at all. For the trio never appeared again, though I have longed to see them many times since that long past summer morning in Denver.

It is very difficult for me to tell of these visions, which I, but nobody else, could see, without seeming to be somewhat demented and having hallucinations.

But they were not like hallucinations at all. They were like something real and yet not real, as though I were seeing something surrounding me from the unseen world. But that sounds strange too. I give up trying to explain them or even convey any real idea as to how they came to me. All I can say is that they were good, and a protection.

On reaching home after this extended American trip I found heaps of letters awaiting me – among them was a little registered parcel containing a present from India. It was from my brother, and sent prior to his war injury. Inside was a brooch showing two larger birds supporting a little bird between them – exactly like those I had seen in my clairvoyant vision.

Was this just a case of coincidence ... or was it a case of mental affinity which had prompted him unconsciously to send me such a brooch as a birthday present? I don't know. All I can say is that it held very special meaning to me.

I never told him how extraordinarily *apropos* his present was. I have always looked upon that brooch as a mascot, and I have worn it ever since.

....

CLINICAL REPORT

End of Session Three. Client/Subject pleasantly aroused from hypnosis following her telling of this phase of her lifetime as Katharine Bates, in search of the mental phase of psychic phenomena. Told exactly as it was recited. Session Four arranged.

For my personal comments on this session, see over ...

PERSONAL NOTATIONS TO MYSELF:

I find myself liking Katharine Bates very much. She is anything but an evangelist trying to convert one to anything. She strikes me as an exceptionally intelligent woman who has a sincere interest in investigating psychic phenomena, for which she herself appears to have a gift.

She is not gullible, yet neither is she closed-minded. Hers is the honest sincere nature of the true investigator who seeks to discover what is true of what she senses in her heart is the true nature of man's status in the universe.

Subject seems to be becoming increasingly articulate in each session. Further, there seems to be developing a sort of subtle connection: blending one personality into the other – as though there is a subconscious recognition each for the other – an understanding that they are both the same soul in ONE.

What has made these continuing sessions with Sarah so outstanding is the flow of continuity which she presents of her time of being such an unusual and interesting person as she was in that lifetime, in pursuing so diligently her investigations of psychic phenomena and spiritualism.

Her story as Katharine Bates continues ...

Chapter Four

THE MANIFESTATIONS OF GEORGE ELIOT

Pre-session Interview. Checked with client about her experiences since her previous session. She said she that she had been very busy and had only had the opportunity to play the tape late in the evening and each time she had fallen asleep. She described it as "Simply the best sleeping pill I have ever taken". She had however listened to the tape just before leaving home that day. She said that she found some of the detail beyond her understanding so we spent a little time talking about psychic matters in general.

This time in order to keep control of Sarah's entry into trance I told her she could not go into trance before I instructed her to do so. When I was ready I gave her the instruction to go into trance and away she went and almost immediately commenced the continuation of her story of Katharine.

Session 4

My next adventure in psychic investigation took me to Australia and New Zealand, following very much the same route which my dear friend, Eleanor, had taken. I sailed shortly after the Jubilee of 1887 had taken place.

My first psychic experience in Australia occurred in Melbourne, some months after my arrival.

The wife of a prominent magistrate in Melbourne had been invited to meet me at an afternoon reception in the house of friends to whom I had letters of introduction, and I was to be introduced to a Mrs. Burroughs, whom I understood was very interested in anything psychic, and would like to hear of my American experiences.

Fortunately the lady arrived late. We had already enjoyed some interesting conversation before she came. A wetter "wet blanket" I have never encountered.   I had heard she was interested in psychic things but, as far as I was concerned, she was disastrously critical. She sat with a cold, glassy eye fixed on me, as I did my best to keep the conversation pleasant.   By this time I had gained something of a reputation in giving clairvoyant readings, so it may well be that she was simply jealous of me.

She might just as well have *said* as she looked at me the words, "Go ahead and make a fool of yourself – that is what I came to see." The position was hopeless, so I began to talk about the weather. Talking about the weather is as good an excuse as anything when conversation is impossible. Presently the daughter of the house came up to me and said, "Do please go on telling us about your psychic experiences in England and America. We can talk of other things at any time, and we had asked Mrs. Burroughs to meet you."

The lady in question had joined another group by this time, so I was able to whisper a reply, "I am sorry, but I cannot possibly talk of these things before that woman – she paralyses me absolutely from the psychic point of view."

"How very odd!" was the unexpected reply. "That is just what my friend, Lizzie Maynard, says. I very much did want Lizzie to hear about America too, but she has gone off to the other end of the room, saying she knows you won't be able to talk while Mrs. Burroughs is here."

This was interesting, for I had not noticed the young girl mentioned, who had not been introduced to me. So, when my hostess asked if she might bring Lizzie to see me at my hotel next day, I gladly acquiesced, in spite of feeling very far from well at that moment.

This feeling of *malaise* increased in the night, and literally made me ill. Being in bed next afternoon about four o'clock, I was dismayed to hear that Miss Maynard had arrived to see me and, moreover, had arrived *alone*. I had never spoken to the girl nor even consciously set eyes on her before, but I knew she must have come at least several miles into the city to make this visit. There was nothing for it, therefore, but to make an effort, order tea to be brought to my room, and send a message hoping she would not mind seeing me in my bedroom.

She came up – a charming girl of about twenty. I explained the circumstances and apologised for being unable to join in the tea party, but felt rather desperate when I realized that even the effort of taking part in a conversation was beyond me.

Suddenly a brilliant idea passed through my throbbing head. The day before, in planning the visit, it had been mentioned that Lizzie Maynard was a very good automatic writer, and this seemed a solution to difficult conversation.

So when the young lady had finished her tea, I said to her, "I am so sorry I am somewhat physically low today. I cannot talk, but I can listen. Do you think you could possibly write a little for me? Our hostess yesterday told me you wrote automatically sometimes."

"I will try, certainly," was the girl's ready response. "I never know, of course, what may come through, but I should like to try."

She found a paper and pencil and sat by my bedside; holding the pencil very loosely between her second and third fingers, instead of between the thumb and first finger in the usual way.

She continued talking to me during the whole time. I could hardly believe that any writing was going on in this very casual way.

"Is any writing coming?" I questioned at last.

"Oh yes, but I can't make out the last long word," she said turning the paper around, so she could read the writing that had come through. "Kindly give me that word again," she remarked, and continued her conversation with me.

The word "miscellaneous" was written, and added to the sheets of calligraphy. She handed the sheets of writing to me.

The whole message was intensely interesting to me, for it began, *"I, who on earth was known as George Eliot ..."*.

Now I had more than once seen, but never spoken to, George Eliot in earth life and, although I admired her genius, as all who read her books are bound to do, there seemed no obvious reason why she should come through to me in particular. Moreover, Lizzie Maynard seemed to know little about the famous author beyond her name.

I searched my memory for any sort of tie with George Eliot that I could think of. I remembered having heard she had often lectured at Oxford on invitation of the dean. As a literary authority she was internationally acclaimed.

Of course there was little chance in those faraway days of my being asked to meet such a brilliant star.

Any friends at Oxford I may have had were but a feeble link. Apparently it now lay with me to cease asking *why*, and accept without question this opportunity to communicate with the spirit of this wonderful person. On such occasions so many possible questions loom up it is difficult to select one with which to start.

At the tea party previously from which I had left with such a headache, there had been some discussion of another woman writer whose books had just begun to reach the zenith of their popularity. I had read one or two, and really had no special opinion about the author. Here was a question to start with.

"What did George Eliot think of the author who was currently being much discussed?"

Very quickly came the answer written on the paper, *"I have no sympathy there – a mere puppet."*

Certainly this was no thought reading, for my own opinions about the matter were very indefinite, and Lizzie had none at all. It was not until some time later that I realised what an extraordinary *apt* criticism had been made – for a puppet is made to dance by other entities rather than by itself.

I put another question, telling Lizzie to ask it in her mind.

"Please ask George Eliot if she *now* thinks she was justified in the position she took with regard to Lewes?"

In a flash the answer came, *"CERTAINLY. We are one here, as we were on earth."*

Amongst other details, George Eliot said finally that she had come to know my mother in spirit life, where she was called STELLA. Now my mother's name in earth life was Ellen, which has the same root for its origin. Of course, Lizzie had no idea as to whether my mother was alive or dead, and certainly knew nothing concerning her Christian name.

The last statement made by George Eliot, in this automatic writing message, was that *before another year had rolled by, a great psychic gift would be bestowed upon me, and I must be very careful to use it without abusing it.* I was too much under-the-weather at the moment to ask whether "another year rolling by" meant a whole year from 28 October 1887 (the date of the message) or the end of the current year, namely, 31 December 1887?

When the message had come to an end, Lizzie Maynard gathered up the scattered sheets and, promising to copy them for me, took her departure, and left me to my own thoughts regarding the curious and interesting result of her visit.

Lizzie! That young lady had proved herself a really remarkable natural medium. In her automatic writing, she held a "key" to unlock one of the doors to the Unseen World.

My next psychic adventure in "The Land Down Under" was about to begin ...

I had come to Australia to join my dear friend, Eleanor Greenleaf, who had been my companion in America, and who had thence sailed for New Zealand and Sydney when I returned for a year to England. She had been anxious for me to rejoin her in Australia, and then go on to visit Japan and China but, my arrival having been delayed, she had finally lost patience and, without my knowledge, had gone to New Zealand, and from there on to Samoa. When I heard of her going to New Zealand I followed her there, on a will-o'-the-wisp expedition as it turned out but, fortunately, I was unaware of this at the time. I say *fortunately* because, had I known that she had already left New Zealand for Samoa, I should certainly have returned to England, giving up trying to trace her any further, and thereby one of my most interesting adventures would have been lost.

My illness in Melbourne was really more serious than I had at first suspected, and it took a fortnight for me to get back on my feet. So the illness seems to have been a factor involved in my next adventure, as I have called it. For the delay led to my meeting – in a friend's house – Mr. Arthur Kitchener (a younger brother of Lord Kitchener) who was introduced to me on the special grounds that we were fellow travellers to New Zealand. As a matter of fact, Mr. Kitchener was on his way from England to New Zealand to supervise some work for his famous brother.

My steamship from Australia to New Zealand was the *Massilia*. Many others were going to New Zealand, but I felt I wanted to be alone, so I kept to the upper deck. Even so, while on the trip, Mr. Kitchener and I became sufficiently friendly for him to give me an invitation to spend the last few days of the year at his "station", about nine miles from Dunback, in the Dunedin district of New Zealand. I must have told him of my disappointment in missing my companion in Sydney, after travelling so many thousand miles to join her and, doubtless, he felt some interest in this "Stanley and Livingstone" sort of chase, with two women taking the principal characters.

Anyway, the invitation was given and accepted, and he kindly promised to ask a couple of his friends to meet me at his house.

All this came to pass some weeks later, on my return from a Bay of Islands trip. This had been a pleasure trip that I took just for the fun of it, and it gave me the opportunity to enjoy that glorious area of New Zealand.

I spent a week at Mr. Kitchener's home and persons there, knowing of my interest in psychic investigation, asked me to conduct an impromptu seance with them. Frankly, I do not like to conduct a seance with no purpose in mind other than curiosity but, as my host wanted it too, I consented. So that Saturday night, 31 December 1887, found me sitting at a table with a few other people, holding a seance in that remote area of New Zealand.

As some reward for any virtue in yielding my point, I suddenly remembered that George Eliot's message, on 28th October, (two months previously), had been: *Before another year had rolled by, a great gift would be bestowed on me, and I must be very careful to use it without abusing it.*

It was almost New Year's Day so, if some message for me was to come through before the rear rolled by, it was now or never, during the few hours still remaining in the current year. I began to give our impromptu seance more serious attention.

After the usual inanities - "I am sure you are pushing"; "I saw your fingers pressing heavily"; "How extraordinary: that is exactly what I thought about you", etc. - suddenly the table became animated by a spirit giving its name as George Eliot. That name coming through brought all the joking to a halt, and our entire group sat at attention.

I put a question to the table, "To what year are you referring?"

"I did not mean another year from October last – I referred to this year," was the answer.

"Shall I write the message automatically?" was my next query.

"No, that is not for you."

"Shall I be able to hear the message? Shall I become clairvoyant?"

"No," came the second time.

My next question naturally was, "Then shall I be able to *see* the message?"

"Yes. Already you have had visions which show you possess talent for the second sight. You are going to become powerfully clairvoyant but, beyond that, you are being given the gift of SEEING THE UNSEEN. Remember my caution for you to use but not abuse the gift."

All the sitters were listening seriously to the message.

"When will it come through?" I asked. The leg of the table rose and fell four times. Mr. Kitchener was the first to speak, "I guess that means that you will see somebody or something during the night or, rather, at four o'clock in the morning."

That ended our little seance, and turned our attention to having some New Year's revelry as midnight announced 1888.

The remarkable point is that I did have an important clairvoyant vision that night, though it had come and gone long before 4.00a.m.

It must be remembered that the dating of the calendar in the southern hemisphere is one day earlier than in my customary northern hemisphere so, to my consciousness, my clairvoyant insight came to me before the old year did roll by, exactly as it was predicted.

Out here, the sun rises at about 3.30a.m. during the end of December and the first week in January, so it would have been fairly light before 4.00a.m. whereas, when I woke out of my sleep that night, my room seemed totally dark. My room was a conventional white-walled apartment, with a wooden bed standing about two or three feet from the wall and parallel with the only window in the room. The window faced the door at the foot of my bed, and was fitted with a heavy, dark green blind on account of the hot summer sunshine.

As I have said, my room was dark. I woke facing the window but turned on my side, and this brought me face to face with the wall. To my infinite amazement there stood, between the wall and my bed, a diaphanous figure of a woman; life size, with one arm held out in a protecting fashion towards me. The figure was faintly luminous so, even in my dark room, I could see her clearly. There seemed to be some form of misty drapery about the head, but the features of the woman were quite distinct and, as I afterwards realised, were the counterpart of photographs I had seen of George Eliot's Savonarola-like countenance. But at the moment only two thoughts came to me: first, how extraordinary was such an apparition; second, how in the world did it happen that I was not the least bit frightened?

I lay there absolutely content and peaceful, with a feeling of blissful satisfaction, and these thoughts passed through my head :-

"Everything is all right – nothing can really ever go wrong – nothing at least that matters at all. All the real things are all right. I can never doubt this truth after this experience. It was promised, and the promise has been redeemed."

Absolutely, those are exactly the thoughts which passed through my head as I lay, fully awake, and looked up at the comforting female figure. It seemed far more than a mere vision. I have spoken of the figure as diaphanous because it was not as solid as an ordinary human being but, on the other hand, I could not see the wall through it; it was too solid for that. I brought to my mind a remembered story, written by a Dr. Jephson, told in the *Athenaeum*, of all papers, of his experience while paying a visit to Lord Offord and making notes for some literary work on hand, late at night, in the library of the house. He had finished his notes, put away the book of reference, looked at his watch, found the hands showing 2.00a.m., (so far as I remember), and had just said to himself, "Well, I shall be in bed by two thirty after all," when, turning round, he found a large leather chair close to his own in which was seated a Spanish priest in some ancient dress!

Thinking it must be an hallucination, he deliberately turned around – away from the priest – rubbed his eyes, and then slowly looked back. Still the priest was there and Dr. Jephson then realised for the first time that, although not *consciously* frightened or alarmed in any way, he was quite unable to speak to the spectral figure. So he picked up a pencil and calmly sketched a portrait of the priest. The priest politely remained until the sketch was completed, and then vanished.

This story, which I had read some years previously, is exactly what flashed through my mind, and I thought, "I will try turning around, and then see if she is still there." I turned deliberately and then turned back again. She was still there. I did see her in fact, although she was impossible in theory. I saw her as distinctly in my dark room as I ever saw a marble statue in the Vatican Gallery by the light of noon. Although I had recalled the Jephson story so circumstantially, it never struck me that it might be interesting to attempt any conversation and see whether I, also, was tongue-tied.

I did *want to speak*, yet there seemed no special need for speaking. It was quite enough to lie there with this blissful feeling of protection and love enshrouding me. And as this consciousness held me in its loving grasp, to my infinite sorrow, this wonderful protecting figure disappeared, gently and very slowly, sinking into the spot in my room where I had first seen her; and once more, all was dark in my room.

I lay peaceful and happy for some ten minutes before it even struck me to check the time. So I lit the candle by my side to find out what o'clock it might be.

Now, I have a rather accurate idea of time and can generally tell within a minute or two how long any special work may have taken me. Looking at my watch I saw it was just 2.25a.m., so I presumed that I must have seen the figure around 2.15a.m. Anyway, I felt sure that ten minutes at least had elapsed between the sinking of the figure out of sight and my lighting the candle in order to consult my watch.

Next morning at breakfast, I told my host and the guests there of my vision. They listened in silent respect, and then Mr. Kitchener said quietly, "Oh yes, you saw something at 4.00a.m. I am not surprised to hear that, as I tried a little psychic experiment of my own at 4.00a.m."

"Not at 4.00a.m.," I answered, "but at 2.15a.m. I carefully checked the time. I was asleep again long before 4.00a.m., and never slept better in my life."

He looked puzzled, and then suggested that my watch must have gone wrong; but we compared our watches, and they matched precisely.

I found out later about the experiment he had tried, having learned something of thought transference theory at a metaphysical club he had attended. He had attempted to make me see a vision at 4.00a.m., but he confessed he had been fast asleep at the time I had seen my vision.

A deeply interesting corroboration reached me a few weeks later, while I was touring interesting places in New Zealand, and had arrived safely at Auckland in the North Island.

I determined to write and ask Lizzie Maynard of Melbourne if she could throw any light on the George Eliot visitation. Several weeks later I received her reply. Her letter went on to state ...

"... I was with a friend that night whom I had told of George Eliot using my hand to convey her message to you last October. My friend asked me to try to contact the spirit of the famous author again. We decided to try it using a planchette. The planchette started to move, then suddenly stopped, and then wrote in bold letters, 'NO. I CANNOT STAY WITH YOU NOW. I HAVE PROMISED TO GO AND SEE STELLA'S DAUGHTER.' I remember, dear Miss Bates, that she had said your mother's name in spirit life was *Stella* so, of course, we knew she was going to see you."

I wrote to Mr. Kitchener of this corroboration of my George Eliot visitation from another source entirely. He reported the manifestation to the Auckland Society of Psychic Research, and the story was printed in their Journal.

....

CLINICAL REPORT

End of Session Four.   Client/Subject pleasantly aroused from hypnosis.   She professed having no recall of the George Eliot experience, yet I did note a certain glow of happiness enter her eyes when that name was mentioned. Session Five arranged.

PERSONAL NOTATIONS TO MYSELF:

I have frequently noticed that there seem to come into every person's lifetime certain events that hold special importance.   This George Eliot episode was of unquestioned importance to the life of Katharine Bates and, as such, was of equal importance to my client, Sarah Channing, in this lifetime.   It seems we all have GUIDES outside, from beyond ourself, who seem to be close by to help us - to give us strength, guidance, protection.   Very possibly that is what is meant by the term, "Guardian Angel".   If that is true, what a wonderful guardian angel George Eliot is for Sarah.

Chapter Five

AN AMAZING SPIRITUALISTIC
EXPERIENCE IN NEW YORK

Pre-session Interview. Checked with client about her experiences since her previous session. All very satisfactory. She had listened to the tape on several occasions. Has obtained a book on spiritualism that I recommended at the last session and is reading it. Client asked many questions relating to the last session but none of particular relevance.

Followed a similar pattern as last time to maintain control over my client as she enters hypnosis. She returned to the story of Katharine Bates almost immediately after I had instructed her to.

Session 5

The spring months of 1888 found me at Brisbane, *en route* for China, after spending a pleasant month with new friends on the estate named Eton Vale, belonging to the late Sir Arthur Hodgson, and situated in the beautiful countryside of Darling Downs in Queensland.

Before returning to Sydney from New Zealand, the girl who had been destined to become my closest friend, Eleanor Greenleaf, reappeared upon the scene in the most unexpected manner. If ever there was a free spirit it was Eleanor. The girl had everything: looks, money and no ambition except to enjoy life. If ever there was the personification of Tilopa's admonition, *"If you would become Enlightened, live life fully to the hilt,"* it was Eleanor. I sometimes call her my female "Dr Livingstone". As I said, she had reappeared unexpectedly upon the scene.

Our "historical meeting" took place in an Auckland hotel, where she suddenly turned up one day, driven back from Samoa by the intense heat. So, after some gentle recriminations (she having supposed that the delay on my part might mean an entire change of plans, and I having supposed, from her letters, that Sydney was such a paradise that she could hardly be dragged from that city even by a flaming sword) we agreed to cry "quits" and continue our travels together. So, Eleanor spent the month of March in Sydney while I paid my visit to Queensland, and we met once more at Brisbane to take a steamer for Thursday Island, Cape Darwin, and eventually Hong Kong. Only one small incident of a psychic nature occurred during this voyage.

You will recall my mentioning my visions of the little "swallows", which I first saw in San Francisco in 1886. And I have had the visitations ever since, causing me to be regarded as a victim of "eye trouble" by some commiserative friends.

On the very day we went aboard the Hong Kong steamer at Brisbane, a new sign appeared to me: a single bird, holding in its beak a ring with a half loop of five glittering diamonds. It came in strongly to my increasing clairvoyant vision: as "George Eliot" had said would be the case, as a gift to me. I told my friend about the vision, but neither she nor I could imagine any significance in it. At that time, we had not even met any of our fellow passengers to speak to, for we were all taken up with settling into our cabins, and trying to make ourselves as comfortable as circumstances would permit.

For the entire following week, the image of the same little bird, holding in its beak a half loop of five glittering diamonds, appeared before my vision. Suddenly an intuition of its meaning hit my consciousness. What the insight was I will tell you just a little later as, within a fortnight of our sailing, the hunch was confirmed. This new (what shall I call it) "sign in the heavens" vanished as soon as I grasped its meaning.

From Brisbane to Hong Kong, from Hong Kong to Japan, nothing of a psychic nature occurred. I must say, however, that Eleanor and I had a delightful time in Japan.

We left Japan eventually, sailing from Yokohama to Vancouver, B.C., and on that part of our journey, something psychicly interesting did occur. We were on board the old P.& O. *Abyssinia*, manned by Captain MacArthur. It is now the *late* Captain MacArthur. He was a kindly and genial naval man, of Australian birth, but belonging to the English Navy, and was just returning home to accept his promotion to Commodore.

On a long steamer trip such as we were on, new acquaintances are quickly made, and confidences shared. I told him of some of my experiences with spirit communication using "the table". The idea intrigued him, so he had the ship's carpenter put together a small, rough wooden table for the *experiment* (as he called it). We tried some "sittings" all together. The sittings were held after dinner with just the three of us present: Eleanor, the Captain and myself. We held our sittings privately in my cabin. For the most part our seance efforts were fruitless, but one incident of real value did occur. My dear old nurse, who tended me so kindly when I was a child, came through (you will recall my mentioning her in telling of my early years while living in Oxford). She had died, and had been on the other side of the veil for some four years. Never before had there been any communication from her but, during our impromptu shipboard seances, she manifested strongly, her message imploring me to give up a proposed tour in Alaska.

Eleanor's and my plans to visit Alaska had never been consummated while we had been in Victoria two years earlier, so she was keen to go there now when we reached Vancouver which, after all, was not too distant. Personally, I was not especially *keen* on making that trip into northern waters, but I had no real objection to it, and it was understood that we should go together.

81

This was the tour which the spirit of my old nurse now pleaded so anxiously for me not to take. Her message ran, *"It will ruin your health, my darling."* She said more than once, *"Don't go there; take my advice."* And on one occasion, just before landing, she added, *"You will find letters awaiting you which will enable you to make other plans."* The messages meant very little to Eleanor and even less to Captain MacArthur. However, to me her messages proved true – in a certain way.

On arriving in Vancouver some letters were awaiting me. One of my letters told of the sudden death of our family solicitor, which would have constituted a good excuse for a hasty return to England, had any such pretext been necessary.

But this was not the case, for my companion, although determined to go to Alaska herself, was not in the least inclined to insist that I accompany her. Eleanor Greenleaf was a very independent woman (which was one of the reasons I liked her so much), and was quite accustomed to travelling alone, and I knew that my decision whether to go to Alaska or not would not affect her going. Frankly, I really did not particularly care to make the trip and thought, very possibly, my old nurse's warning might be justified. However, I shrugged it off, and decided to accompany my friend to Alaska. As things turned out, I probably made the right decision, although my nurse's earnest entreaties were only too fully justified on the physical plane; to say nothing of the miserable discomfort of the trip (which, in those days, had to be made in an overcrowded cargo boat). I took on a serious cold in those Arctic regions, which later developed into one of the most serious illnesses I ever had in my life. It took months to make even a partial recovery, and definitely weakened my lungs. Yet, I never regretted my decision.

This episode taught me a great deal as to how spirit messages should be taken. They should be held as opinions, and are not to be regarded as infallible predictions. They can be looked upon as advice and warnings, but how they are accepted and acted upon is entirely up to the recipient. In other words, we must judge for ourselves; we cannot shift the burden of responsibility on to any other shoulders – spirit or otherwise. That is a universal lesson for us all.

Had I turned my back on Alaska, I should have gained enormously, physically speaking, and yet missed out on witnessing one of the most amazing spiritualistic demonstrations of my life. My dear old nurse was only considering dangers to my health to be avoided.

As a result of my prolonged illness, Eleanor and I had once again to be separated. She was obliged to return to England alone, while I remained in a Canadian hospital.

I knew I had to get well as rapidly as I could and return to England. Finally, my physician certified that I was in good enough condition to undertake the voyage. En route I spent two days in New York, and it was while there that I was met by a Dr. Theodore Covernton, and I persuaded this gentleman to accompany me to a seance held by Mrs. Stoddard Gray.

Dr. Covernton had all the conventional prejudices that a staid man of medicine usually has. However, he was intelligent and open-minded enough to discuss such subjects as hypnotism and psychic phenomena. I commented that for a physician to resist all such mental aids would be to miss out on some valuable adjuncts to his profession. He was reasonable enough about it. Anyway, we ended up attending a seance together, and he accompanied me to the home of Mrs. Stoddard Gray, the well-known New York medium of whom I have spoken before.

The usual performance of devotional singing and requests for spirit guidance went on, but nothing occurred that was really of interest to Dr. Covernton or myself. Then an incident took place which amazed him, an occurrence so startling that it defied explanation, and it happened in full light – right at our very feet.

A gentleman and a lady who were sitting in the circle had brought with them their little boy, a child of seven years old. I asked the mother if the seance wasn't keeping the boy up rather late, and her answer was cheerful and good-natured:

"Well, I guess we wouldn't have much peace at home if we didn't bring Edgar along with us to the seance to see his Granny. We brought him once, and since then he always insists on coming. He loves talking to his Granny."

At this moment, a small, frail woman stepped out from the cabinet and came right towards us, motioning to the little grandson that she wanted him to go into the cabinet with her. This he did without a moment's hesitation. The curtain fell and concealed them both from view. What happened within the cabinet I do not know but, some minutes later, when the little boy reappeared, he was holding Granny by the hand and seemed very happy. Then occurred one of the most amazing spirit manifestations I have ever witnessed. Even now, as I tell about it, I can scarcely believe it, but I'll swear on any number of Bibles this is exactly what happened:

The child had brought some toys – a little wooden train and some building blocks – "to get Granny to play with him as usual", and the fragile old lady knelt down on the floor and played with him, just as any ordinary Granny might have done.

In the very midst of their having fun together, something occurred which caused the little boy to burst into tears. Granny had evidently forgotten that her time on this plane was limited, by conditions of which we are still profoundly ignorant.

Quite suddenly, and without a word of warning, she disappeared: not into the cabinet at her back, but right through the carpet under our feet, and within a yard of where we were seated. It was an instant dematerialization. One moment the old lady was there; the next she had disappeared into a cloud of mist, and even this was quickly withdrawn, apparently through the floor. It was beyond startling; it was positively uncanny. Dr. Covernton dropped to his knees and pounded the carpet where she had disappeared. This was no trickery; just solid carpeting, covering a solid floor. There was simply no explanation for what had happened other than spirit dematerialization.

As I have said, when his Granny disappeared so suddenly the child burst into tears and his parents had to take Edgar away, still sobbing. His parents said they had taken him to the seances here many times to meet Granny, and nothing like this had ever happened before.

The medium, Mrs. Stoddard Gray, was very indignant about it and spoke tartly, "Too bad! She ought to have *known* she was staying too long, and risking a fright to the child. If only she had gone back into the cabinet he would not have been frightened. But she stayed too long and did not have enough strength to hold her form."

I had a clairvoyant flash at that moment: that the little boy, Edgar, was the power through which Granny managed to materialize so well and that, when he grew up, he would be acclaimed as one of the greatest psychics the world has ever known.

That clairvoyant gift of having insight about future events was the meaning, it had come to me, symbolized by the five glittering diamonds held in the loop in the little bird's mouth: The five flashes – each a diamond of advanced perception.

This ability of the mind to know of events prior to their occurring is one of the great mysteries of psychic phenomena. I don't profess to fully understand it; I just know it is so.

It was a very puzzled and quiet Dr. Theodore Covernton who escorted me back to my hotel. I never saw the man again.

Well, I ask you, was my suffering in Alaska worth this absolutely phenomenal experience? It was a once in a lifetime event, which I would have missed out completely had my timing not been exactly as it was.

I think I made the right decision.

....

CLINICAL REPORT

End of Session Five.   Sarah pleasantly aroused from hypnosis. Amnesia. Session Six arranged.

PERSONAL NOTATIONS TO MYSELF:

As I work with this client, helping her recapture her memories of experiences in her previous lifetime as Katharine Bates ... each session makes me realize more and more how truly limited are the normal senses of man. There are things he cannot see; things he cannot hear; things he cannot feel; things he cannot smell; things he cannot taste.

These sessions have made me appreciate what a wonderful UNIVERSE we exist in.

These sessions have even seemed to activate more my own glimpses into the unseen world.

The more I experience SEEING THE UNSEEN, the more fully alive I *realize* we all truly are.

I now await with great interest what adventures will be described in Session Six.

Chapter Six

PSYCHIC EXPERIENCES IN INDIA

Pre-session Interview. Checked with client about her experiences since her previous session. Nothing particular to report. Client has now settled into a comfortable rhythm, does what I suggest. Seems to fully accept that we may well have many more sessions to come and we can only go at a pace that is right for her. Client also seems to want to spend more time in between sessions in attempting to understand all the content of the tapes. Her thirst for knowledge is truly prodigious.

Client went into trance as soon as she lay back on the couch and after a short pause returned to her story of Katharine.

Session 6

My psychic experiences in India were of a very personal nature.

In the month of November 1890 I set off, with my friend Eleanor, on my first visit to India. My companion was still at the age where social India was naturally more interesting to her than either the historical or mystical aspects of the country. As for myself, I went there on my initial trip more to see the glorious temples of a magnificent past than with any view of learning any occult secrets from the Fakirs and Yogis of the present.

Under Great Britain's dominion, many Hindus seem to look upon the British in general as being materialistic, without much room for the mystical in their souls. Personally, although I am British, there has always been plenty of room for the mysterious and mystical in my soul. Actually, I related extremely well to that magical land.

Nevertheless it took some doing before things "opened up" for me there. From the Indian point of view, a devout and educated Hindu would no more think of discussing his transcendental ideas with an English person than we would think of discussing delicate questions of art with a village yokel. This was confirmed by my noticing the difference in the welcome accorded a charming young Swedish lady, whom we met at Benares on her wedding tour. She had brought excellent native introductions from her own country, where certain Rajahs and Maharajas had been entertained by her King and, thanks to these and, as she said, *"to the fact of my not being English"*, she had access to many interesting places and took part in special functions from which most of us were debarred. However, India is not called "The Land of Magic" for nothing. It goes far beyond the clever conjuring of the Fakirs who may be found by the tourist on every hotel veranda, anxious to pick up a few rupees. There seems to be an actual energy in that country that is conducive to occult experiences.

Making the usual tour, but including Lahore – where my brother had lived at Government House for several years as Military Secretary to Sir Robert Egerton (who was in *his* day Lieutenant Governor of the Punjab) – we came in due course to Delhi.

Our first day there was devoted to tracing Mutiny relics of all kinds and, around 4.00 p.m., we drove out to see the famous Mutiny Memorial. This, as you possibly know, is a red sandstone tower with a staircase of rough stone inside and small windows pierced through at varying intervals. It stands upon an extensive marble flooring, which is inscribed with the names of the officers and men of various regiments who took part in the renowned siege, and died for their country in consequence.

As we drove towards the Memorial, the whole place seemed to be in a flutter of excitement. Hundreds of natives were flocking around, and we both remarked how much more interested they appeared to be in these monuments of past events than the corresponding class of

English labourers would have been. But on arrival we found it was not a question of historical interest. The fact was that a poor native – who had just climbed up the Memorial Tower by the inner staircase – had fallen out of one of the windows, and was lying on the marble floor below at the far side from us, crushed and dying. We were told that an Englishman had, fortunately, been present and had gone off to find a doctor. So nothing could be done for the poor man until the physician arrived.

Meanwhile, our native guide – Bobajee – had rushed off to see what was to be seen of the tragedy and, rather to my horror, my girl companion seemed about to follow his example! It was terrible to think of the poor man lying there in his death agony; but he was already surrounded by natives, and no real help could be given without fear of doing more harm than good before the doctor came. Just to be there and look on without being able to help added extra horror to the tragedy for me. I turned to my young friend who had seemed ready to go off, but she did *not* go. I mention this incident to explain my emotional state, which proved to be a factor in the psychic experience that occurred.

One of my dearest friends in London, who shared my interest in psychic things, was Lady Wincote. We had developed a close rapport. It turned out that she was resting on a couch, following a disturbed night, at the very hour of my visit to the Mutiny Memorial.

It was about noon in England; she was fully awake and had been reading. Looking at her watch she realised it was time to go down for luncheon. Suddenly the door opened and *I* walked into her resting room and around the couch upon which she was reclining, until I stood between her and the window, which was to her left.

I appeared to be dressed in outdoor attire, and seemed much excited about something. I was talking continuously as it seemed to her, but my sentences were disjointed. She found that she "wondered what had upset me so". She spoke to me, asking what had happened, but she said that I took no notice of her questions and just stood there, standing with my face to the window and my back to her. Then, she said, I turned around and deliberately retraced my steps past the ottoman, skirting around the couch, and was just disappearing through the door when she made a final effort to attract my attention, asking a question:

"Kathy! Tell me before you go, what number are you staying at in Oxford Terrace?" (the part of the city where I always stayed at that time of year). Lady Wincote said, "You made no answer at all, but whisked out of the door in a great hurry and then, for the first time, I remembered *that you were in India.* It had all seemed so natural, as you have often been in my home, and I thought for the moment that you must have returned unexpectedly to London. My one anxiety was to know which number the Terrace would find you, in case you had changed your address."

This was truly a profound psychic experience, which was subsequently collaborated, as Lady Wincote wrote to me about it on the very day that it occurred, i.e. 8 January 1891; and her letter crossed with mine telling of the incident. I have a complete record of the event, corresponding with the date of Lady Wincote's letter to me. (Subsequently I reported this psychic manifestation to the London Society of Psychic Research, as an out-of-body experience.)

Further to this incident, was a conversation I had with Bobajee. I was looking inside the Memorial, and had seen that the stone steps were crumbling away and looked very unsafe. He said to me, "Something bad there, Lady Sahib." I concluded that he was referring to the state of the staircase, and attributed the poor native's fall to some such cause.

But he denied this strenuously, *"No! No! Lady Sahib ... some bad devil inside there. He threw boy over!"*

Then Bobajee went on to tell us that on one special night in the year no native man, woman or child in the whole city could be induced to pass the Mutiny Memorial at midnight. The few daring persons who *had* passed there had found the tower lighted up inside, and the sepoys and the British soldiers had come back, and were fighting their battles all over again! The man assured me that all Delhi people knew this to be a fact, and gave the place a wide berth on that anniversary.

The idea of a "bad devil" throwing the poor boy down from the top of the tower, followed by this curious legend, interested me as a bit of folklore, but my girl companion was almost scornful. "Silly nonsense, Bobajee!" was her sarcastic reception of the story, and this made me feel intensely sorry that Lady Wincote, who would have been as interested as myself, should not have been present. Did this moment of intense desire for her project itself into the appearance she saw in her room? Certainly it was a remarkable coincidence that she should see me obviously feeling emotionally disturbed, so many thousands of miles away.

It was one of the most remarkable examples of spontaneous astral projection I have ever come across. *And it was my own.*

I had another profound psychic experience on the very day succeeding that last event, that chilled me to the bone.

My companion being slightly ill, I had driven out alone with our native guide. We made a long tour around Ludlow Castle, of the famous Mutiny memory, and still, in the year 1891, a Government bungalow.

The present Czar of Russia was travelling through India at the time as Czarevitch with his cousin Prince George of Greece, and they were expected to arrive in Delhi that same evening. The royal party were to be lodged at Ludlow Castle. They were expected within the hour.

Bobajee jumped off the box of my carriage and urged me to, "Go, look see!"

"No, Bobajee! Drive on – I can't go look see – they will not let me in."

"Yes, yes, Lady Sahib," he said eagerly, "everything ready – all gone away – nobody in there yet."

This seemed inconceivable, but it proved to be absolutely true. I went in, expecting to be turned back before I had crossed the hall, but there was no one there! The place was like a City of the Dead. Yet within an hour a banquet arranged for about seventy people was to take place. I made an examination of the place and went through numerous bedrooms. At length I went into the dining room – a long narrow room – arranged for the coming banquet. At least sixty to seventy table settings were laid; flowers arranged on the table cloth in artistic Indian fashion and all the beautiful glass and silver placed in readiness.

Nothing was missing but the presence of the guests for whom all this preparation had been made.

The short Indian twilight was already upon us as I stood there for a moment, contrasting the dead and almost eerie silence with the lights and laughter that would soon replace it.

A fireplace was close to me as I stood at the far end of the room, looking down the whole length of the table. Glancing up, I realised that the only picture in the room was hung over this fireplace. The picture had no great artistic value; the painting was poorly done. It was a badly drawn portrait of a man about thirty five years of age, with long whiskers. It looked old, and I guessed it probably had been done by the poor artist possibly thirty or forty years previous to my visit.

But as I looked carefully at it, a curious sensation came over me. There was something in the eyes of the portrait that held me; something that rose triumphant above the artist's limitations. At the same moment, I was conscious of a Presence behind my back, *of somebody who was looking at the picture with me,* of somebody who was giving an inner message to my psyche, *"That is a picture of me, but I am not there – I am here, close to you; behind your shoulder I am looking at it with you."*

The impression was so strong that it seemed almost as if a hand were pressing on my shoulder. I turned around involuntarily, but no one was there. I was alone in the room, yet I was not alone.

Can I possibly convey what I mean?

Then I looked at the picture again, and the impression remained that the man whom the picture represented had been strong enough to make me feel his actual presence in the room, although I could see nothing. There was no name on the picture of either subject or artist, no possible clue to identity and, looked at as a picture alone, there was nothing about it that was outstanding, nothing to account for my feelings.

I could scarcely tear myself away from the almost overwhelming sense of the *presence* of so strong and magnetic a personality, but the fading twilight signalled that I had better make an exit.

As I left the dining room, I went hurriedly through a large and handsome drawing room, which filled with portraits, chiefly of deceased governors and generals, many of them admirably painted, and a striking contrast to the poorly painted picture mounted above the fireplace.

Later, when I told my companion about my experience, she told me that I was imagining things. However, in spite of her passing it off so lightly, I resolved to make inquiries.

"I am going to clear this up!" I said to myself with determination and, in a few days, my perseverance was rewarded, and my impression justified, by finding that I had been looking at the portrait – feeble and poor as it was – of *Brigadier General Nicholson.*

If ever a dead man, who had lived in India, could impress himself as devotedly upon the living of that country, Nicholson would be the man capable of such a feat.

Even to this day there is a religious sect in India called Nicholsonism who have handed down the memory of this "God rather than man", who had to dismount from his horse occasionally to thrash the would-be worshippers, and put a stop to their inconvenient adoration.

Nicholson's brilliant achievements in the Mutiny, his absolute control over men of the most diverse character, the devotion with which he inspired his soldiers, and his own glorious death at the very moment of victory – all these are matters of history.

I am grateful to have known, even for a few passing moments, what that influence in Ludlow Castle's dining room had been and, when I located Brigadier General Nicholson's grave at Delhi after my mystical experience before his portrait, I placed flowers on the grave of an honoured acquaintance, rather than of a man known to me only through history.

I left India with my friend, leaving us, especially myself, with a deep respect for the magic that can occur in "The Land of Magic".

CLINICAL REPORT

End of Session Six. The actual trance session was relatively short compared to previous sessions. This is because Sarah seemed reluctant to continue once she had completed the telling of her experiences in India. However, Sarah pleasantly aroused from hypnosis with complete amnesia for the events that she had recounted as Katharine Bates in India. Session 7 arranged.

PERSONAL NOTATIONS TO MYSELF:

Some of the things this client relates are almost beyond belief. But who is to say? Psychologically it is known that the subconscious can conjure up dreams, often fantasies. On the other hand, the memory bank of the subconscious mind can be detailed and accurate on what it reports. As a hypnotherapist, it is not within my prerogative to judge on the memory-stories that come forth. My position is entirely to induce a proper mental state for such buried memories to flow, via the process of Past Life Hypnotherapy.

Beyond question, what the client is telling of her lifetime as Katharine Bates is fascinating. My responsibility is to accurately record her recounting. I look forward to her continuing in our next session, Sarah as Katharine.

Chapter Seven

SPOOKY ADVENTURES IN RUSSIA

Pre-session Interview. Checked with client about her experiences since the last session. As usual she had played the tape a number of times. She said that she had been to India several times in this life time although she had not visited the same places as Katharine. She said that whilst she had been in India she had had many fleeting feelings of *déjà vu* which at the time she had found a little disturbing. We talked about this for a while and also about the book she had read on spiritualism.

She told me she had bought a book by a fellow member of the National Guild of Hypnotists, Henry Leo Bolduc, entitled "The Journey Within" which is about past lives. I advised her not to start experimenting on too many levels at once but to finish her telling of the story of Katharine and then to look further, and that Henry's book was not a bad place to start. She seemed happy with this approach.

Once on the couch she relaxed instantly into trance and following my signal continued with her story of Katharine.

Session 7

My next personal psychic adventures took place in Russia. They began with a ghost story I was told in Sweden.

I travelled to Sweden in the spring of 1892, and carried with me an introduction to the Swedish Consul at Gothenburg. While in that city I had the good fortune to attend a consulate party and met Mr. and Mrs. Romilly. Mr. Romilly was an Englishman who had married a Swedish lady. We enjoyed several visits together and, knowing of my interest in psychic things, Mr. Romilly told me the story of his first cousin (a well-known lady of title) and her Egyptian necklace. It seemed that it was a present given to her on her marriage, a very ancient and exquisite necklace, with blue stones of a shade well known to travellers in Egypt, and much sought after.

It must have been a genuine article, for she told a tale that one night the ghost of an Egyptian Pharaoh appeared to her and said that the necklace had been rifled from his tomb, and warned her that she would have no peace as long as she persisted in wearing the necklace.

So the lady very wisely locked up the necklace in her home safe, and trusted that the Egyptian ghost would be satisfied.

Not a bit of it! For he appeared again and told her that she would be haunted by his unwelcome presence so long as the necklace *remained in her possession.*

So she took the necklace and deposited it with her lawyer, who locked it in a strong-box in his office, doubtless with a secret smile at his client's superstitions.

But nemesis lay in wait for him as well, and the last thing Mr. Romilly had heard was that the lawyer himself was made so exceedingly uncomfortable by the attentions of the Egyptian spectre that he was obliged to bury the necklace in his back yard. A "score" for the ghost!

It was the kind of spirit and/or ghost story that I found interesting, so I appreciated his telling it to me. However one hears all kinds of stories about Egyptian ghosts coming back and reclaiming treasures taken from their tombs. Whether it was true or not, I had not the slightest idea.

Anyway to cut the story short, while having tea in Gothenburg I met the lady who was the cousin of Mr. Romilly, and I alluded discreetly to the story of the blue necklace.

She said that it was absolutely true, and was not in the least annoyed that her cousin had mentioned it to me. It opened up some good conversation between us, which ended with the comment that if I really wanted to run into some interesting psychic experiences, I should give Russia a try. Slavic people she said are gifted in all sorts of gypsy lore.

So, from Gothenburg I went to Stockholm, and from Stockholm on to St. Petersburg, in which city I had my first new psychic adventures since returning from India.

I telegraphed Eleanor and she joined me for the trip. She was a great travelling companion and, while not overly interested in psychic things, she respected my interest (most of the time), and we had a lot of fun together. In a way, you might say, she was a good balance for me and kept me from getting carried away too quickly.

While in St. Petersburg, we engaged a German named Kuntze. He had lived there for nearly half a century, so was an excellent guide. We were staying at the *Hotel de France*, and Kuntze told us that a celebrated French modiste had taken rooms in our hotel to display her beautiful Parisian creations and take orders from the Russian Royal Family and Ladies of the Court. He also mentioned the Frenchwoman's recent misfortune, in learning – since her arrival in Russia – that her manager in Paris had fled France along with 100,000 francs of her business income.

Two nights later I had gone to bed as usual and must have slept for nearly four hours when I awoke, feeling the heat oppressively. Getting out of bed to open my window still further, I gazed down upon the courtyard, noting the absolute stillness of the hotel and the hot, moist air outside.

Suddenly this stillness was broken by horrible shrieks. Peal after peal rang out. It was ghastly and blood-curdling. For a moment it seemed that I *must* be dreaming. What horrors, to justify such awful shrieks, could have occurred at this quiet hour and in this quiet and respectable hotel?

Nothing less than murder suggested itself to me, and I dashed across my room to check the lock on my door. My next thought was for my companion, Eleanor Greenleaf. She was sleeping in an adjacent room, with a connecting door between us.

I hammered loudly on this, and she finally awoke and opened it as I shouted, "Someone is being murdered out there!"

She said sleepily, "Stop it, Kathy, You're dreaming. I'm sleeping."

I heard other doors in the hotel hallway opening, so I peeked out. Several scared people had poked out their heads. By now the horrible screams had ceased, so the poked out heads withdrew.

My room was a corner one. Exactly opposite my door, with a wide passage between, was the room which had been pointed out to me as being occupied by the famous French modiste.

As I looked down the dimly lit hallway, I spotted a Russian waiter. I beckoned to him and, very reluctantly, he came to my door.

I knew by the way the man shied away from my questioning that he knew more about the matter than he was saying, so I dismissed him impatiently with a sarcastic comment, "What is the good of telling me such nonsense. I know those screams meant far more than a headache. I will find out for myself tomorrow."

The Russian waiter left quickly.

I shut and locked my door, and restlessly lay for an hour or two thinking over the ghastly disturbance, and wondering who the victim might be? It was now 5.00a.m. Dawn was breaking. However, as so often happens even after the most sleepless night, I dozed off then. During my sleep I dreamed – this was my dream:

It must be first noted that there was a wide staircase close to my corner room which continued upward to the next floor. In my dream or vision, I distinctly saw a woman in a white nightgown, with dark hair streaming down her back, rushing up this flight of stairs in the most distraught and reckless fashion. In her hand she held a knife, and was trying to stab herself with it, as the Russian waiter endeavoured to wrench it out of her hand. Two or three people ran up the stairs behind her, but only the Russian waiter seemed to have the courage to grapple with her.

In a few moments it seemed to me that the vision that had entered my mind so startling and so clear faded away, and I sank into a dreamless sleep, and it was close to 8.00a.m. when I woke finally.

When the Russian waiter appeared with my breakfast, I said rather curtly to him, "You need not have troubled to make up that foolish story last night. I know what happened – *I have seen it.*"

He looked incredulous, so I went on, "The lady was trying to kill herself, and rushed up to the next floor with a knife in her hand. I saw you run after her, and force it from her."

The man was speechless. He said not one syllable, either of corroboration or denial, but left the room as quickly as possible looking scared, and certainly left the impression upon my mind that my vision or dream, whatever it was, represented what had actually taken place.

To my surprise however, our dependable German guide, Kuntze, gave a rather different version of the story.

Eleanor had come to my room to join me by then, so he spoke to us both, and at once referred to the terrible tragedy.

"Ah, poor lady! You remember my telling you about her the other day, and how her manager had run away with all the money? Now *this* frightful misfortune has happened to her, and no one knows if she will survive. She is still alive, and is to be taken to the hospital."

Eleanor just stood there looking on indifferently. "But what happened, Kuntze?" I said impatiently, rather irritated by his mysterious allusion, and by Eleanor's apparent indifference. However, as it seemed that she had slept through the whole thing, I could scarcely expect much reaction now. Kuntze's version was far better than the waiter's, and was interwoven with shreds of truth, as I discovered later.

He said the "poor lady" was in the habit of making herself a cup of tea in the middle of the night when wakeful; also that she wore white crepe sleeves on her night attire. She lit a little burner to warm her tea and the sleeve caught fire, and in a few moments she was enveloped in flames, owing to the flimsy material she wore. Then the shrieks began which had so chilled our nerves. A Russian gentleman, sleeping in the next room down the hall, was awakened by her screams and, knowing that she was a rich woman who had brought many valuables with her, concluded that she was being murdered, so he rushed to the rescue with a revolver, found the burning woman and, with the help of the waiter, at length succeeded in putting out the flames.

The story seemed logical but Eleanor shrugged, and could not resist pointing out how entirely it annihilated my dream vision. I love her dearly but she is a minx and, every so often, she will put in a few digs about my being overly sensitive to ascribing psychic interpretations to things. She said, "See: No suicide! No knife! No rushing up the staircase! No nothing at all that you described! All just a figment of your imagination!" I didn't feel so sure she was right but, in the face of Kuntze's explanation, I said nothing and so the matter rested.

The famous French woman remained in the hospital, and her son and daughter were telegraphed for from Paris. We found them at the hotel three weeks later, on our return there from Moscow. There was some slight hope of ultimate recovery but, within six or seven weeks following the "accident", the unfortunate lady died.

From Russia we returned to Stockholm, where Eleanor and I parted for a time. She took the steamer for Hull and I went up into the Dovre Feld Mountains to join Mrs Romilly, whom I have mentioned before.

I told her my story of the poor French *modiste* and her sad and painful accident, and also about my curiously vivid and yet inaccurate vision, and we discussed the matter together. We were then in a remote part of the Dovre Feld, where foreign papers were practically unobtainable.

I had left my friend in Norway and returned to England a week or two before receiving a very interesting letter from her. In it she said, "I have just got hold of some French papers, and I see the poor woman you told me about who died in St. Petersburg has caused quite a news sensation, as she was very well known. The real story has now come out.

"It seems that it was suicide after all, so your vision was quite true!

"She had received large sums in advance for commissions from the Russian nobility, and had either spent or speculated with them. That was why she had to invent the story of an embezzling manager to cover her own shortcomings.

"But the truth leaked out in spite of her trying to keep things hidden, so she made up her mind to commit suicide rather than face the horrors of a Russian prison. The paper goes on to say that she chose a most horrible death. It seems she waited until the middle of the night you described, and then covered her whole body with oil from a lamp in the room, and set fire to herself. That accounts, of course, for the horrible shrieks you heard. In her agony she seized a knife and rushed out into the hallway in a blaze, and when the Russian waiter tried to stop her she ran from him, and attempted to stab herself as she made her way up the stairs. All this you seem to have seen accurately in your dream vision; also the fact that the waiter pursued her and succeeded in wrenching the knife from her hands before she injured herself with it. The paper mentions that a Russian gentleman had gone to the rescue when he heard the shrieks, but this was before she had got hold of the knife, and it was the waiter, alone, who saved her in the end from immediate death."

I know there is a "law of parsimony" which says that when anything is uncertain it is best to accept the simplest explanation but, as my life has proceeded, more and more I have come to appreciate that my psychic perception is more accurate than "the law of parsimony".

During this Russian visit Eleanor and I had gone down to Moscow from St. Petersburg and here again a curious psychic adventure befell me.

It was the height of summer in Russia and we were thankful that each of us had a large, handsome room, with three windows looking over the square and a view of the famous Kremlin in the distance.

My room was divided into two parts, separated by a door which was, during the hot season, thrown wide open and *fastened back securely*. Between this door and the one opening into the outer corridor stood the wash basin, and also a wardrobe cupboard, with a very poor lock on it, as I discovered later.

On retiring the first night I locked the outer door, undressed in this anteroom and finally hung up my clothes in the wardrobe that I have mentioned. Then, after looking out of the window at the crowd below in the square, which had diminished as the night advanced, I went to bed. I felt cheerful and looked forward to having a good rest, as I was very tired from our journey from St. Petersburg to Moscow.

However, as so often happens when one is overtired, sleep did not come. I tried "counting sheep", but in vein. The more I tried to go to sleep, the more restless I became. The midnight hour struck, then the half hour, and I gathered from the stillness below that most of the people in the square had retired to their homes. Then one o'clock struck, and after that I lay for what seemed an eternity before the 1.30a.m. chime sounded. Scarcely had the "bong" ceased when I heard cautious sounds in the corridor, and I heard the outer door of my room being quietly opened. It creaked a little on old hinges. I felt a chill of fear pass up my spine. The thought flashed through my mind that I must not have locked it; yet I knew I had. The best I could hope was that some new arrival had mistaken his room, was returning late and consequently was trying to be as quiet as possible so as not to awaken other residents.

This thought flashed through my mind, and it did help calm my sense of fear a bit. I expected to see a *man's* head appear at the door he had mistakenly opened near the foot of my bed, to hear a hurried apology, and then a hasty retreat. I bunched the covers up around my breasts, and waited for the mistaken intruder to appear. But no one appeared. Several moments passed in horrible suspense for me. The outer door had creaked on its hinges and opened, without a shadow of doubt, *but where was the man?*

The door had not closed again, so far as I could tell. I glanced about the room – there was nobody there. There was nothing but the wash-stand and wardrobe there. But somebody had just entered, and I even recalled muffled footsteps following the creaking of the hinges. Where was the intruder hiding? What could he be *waiting for?* My comforting supposition of a mistaken room vanished – it could not account for the long pause. Perhaps it was a burglar who had entered, and was waiting to be sure his entrance had not been heard before beginning to search for items to steal.

This seemed the only reasonable supposition, and I lay in absolute terror for some minutes, fearing almost to breathe, and quite incapable of putting an end to my terrible suspense. I longed to hear the clock strike again, but nothing relieved the dead silence in my room. At last the friendly tones of the clock struck the "quarter". Somehow it released the tension and gave me courage - the courage of desperation - to strike a match and light my candle. I could see a little about the room now as the darkness receded. The middle door was fastened back, as I had found it. But this was not the door which had been opened; that sound had come from the *outer* door. I knew there was no point in my lying there shivering, so I cautiously got out of bed, tossed on a robe, knew that I must relock the *outer* door and that I must find out if anyone was hiding in my room. I passed through the open *inner* door with fear and trembling. To my relief, the small anteroom was apparently empty. The wardrobe stood partly open, but there was nothing more important in it than a few clothes I had hung up. Then I made my way to the outer door, which opened into the corridor, determined to make sure it was securely locked this time.

I have seldom been more absolutely dumbfounded than when I turned the handle of that door, preparatory to locking it, and found that it was *securely locked already.* How could the hinges have creaked then, and whose cautious footsteps had I heard?

Once more, my eyes fell upon the wardrobe with its cheap lock. I knew I had certainly not locked this, so possibly it was that door which had sprung open and had creaked. I did not for the moment conjecture that the noise had come from another quarter, and that the footsteps were still to be explained. I was only thankful to have given myself this supposed explanation. So I locked the wardrobe as carefully as possible, put out my candle and went back to bed. I felt relieved.

I was almost asleep when the whole scene was repeated again! The same cautious tread; the same creaking sounds as the outer door opened on its rusty hinges. The human mind is funny sometimes: instead of feeling fearful this time, it put me in a defiant mood. My impatience got the better of my fears. I was not going to be decoyed out of bed a second time on a wild-goose chase. Soft footsteps, creaking door opening, a faulty lock on the wardrobe. To heck with it all. I turned on my side and fell into a deep sleep, after the varied excitements of the night.

Next morning I got up feeling remarkably refreshed. I dressed and tested my theory that the whole incident was probably based on that faulty lock on the wardrobe door. To my perplexity, *the wardrobe door was still locked*, just as I had left it in the middle of the night. A mystery. However, I had not been harmed, so I let it stand as an unexplained mystery. However, I did change my room, and took another room at the rear of the hotel, away from the square.

I told Eleanor about what had happened. She showed far more interest in my new adventure than in the St. Petersburg tragedy and so-called vision of mine.

Openly, Eleanor is sceptical of psychic experiences but, underneath, I suspect she is quite psychic. Perhaps that is why we have developed such a good friendship. Surprisingly even to herself, under my instruction she has shown a good talent for automatic writing. "I do it just for fun," she says. Anyway, since she seemed to take an interest in my bedroom experience, I asked her to see what automatic writing might bring out. She is a practical kind of girl, so I knew that what came through would not be based on just imagination. Automatic movements of her hand wrote this message in answer to my question about the night's mystery:

"About fifty years back in time, a Russian officer and his mistress had occupied this large front room in the hotel. This man had spent all day at a rifle competition, combined with some partying, and returned at 1.30a.m. very drunk. He had opened the door to the room very carefully hoping he would find the lady asleep but unfortunately she was not only wide awake, but extremely annoyed by his late return in a state of intoxication. A desperate quarrel had ensued and, getting frightened by his violence, she seized his rifle and gave him a blow on the head with the butt end of it, hoping to stun him, but with no idea of murder in her mind. However, the blow proved fatal – to her extreme remorse."

From this insight, it would seem I had experienced in that hotel in Moscow a ghostly manifestation. Under such circumstances it would seem that it would be the lady who haunted the room, and not the man. However, from my studies of hauntings, it does seem that the energy of the victim returns more often than does that of the perpetrator of the murder.

All I can say as regards the authenticity of this case is to give my personal experience of the haunting that night in my hotel room as I have described it, and Eleanor's automatic writing insight. It was obviously impossible to get a full corroboration of the story. However checking did turn up the facts that the particular hotel we were in had been in existence as far back as fifty years, and also that rifle competitions had taken place during those far off days. Even with some understanding of what it was, if my personal feelings stand for anything, I can definitely say it was a very eerie experience. It still gives me goosebumps!

....

CLINICAL REPORT

End of Session Seven.   Client aroused on my instruction feeling perfectly relaxed with complete amnesia regarding the content of the session.   This session was one of the longest so far. This was primarily due to some long pauses in the client's relating of the experiences.   At times it seemed that she was having to listen very intently indeed but I have no clue as to what she was listening for or to. Client as usual looking forward to the next session.

PERSONAL NOTATION TO MYSELF:

One thing I have observed about hypnotic behavior is that the more frequently the subject uses the state, the more natural it seems to appear as objective behavior.   Very much is this the case in the Sarah/Katharine regression. I especially wish to keep each personality distinct from the other.   I do not fear integration, but such must be under volitional control.

Session Eight arranged.

Chapter Eight

A-HAUNTING WE WILL GO

Pre-session interview. Carried out the usual checks and everything appeared normal. Much of the pre-session discussion was devoted to the subject of ghosts and whether or not they are spirits trapped between one life and the next and how they can be helped to move on to their next incarnation. Obviously Sarah is learning quite a lot from her studies in spiritualism and from the content of her regressions to the the time when she was Katharine.

As soon as Sarah lay down on the couch she relaxed and rapidly entered a deep trance and following my signal continued with her story of Katharine.

Session 8

In the autumn of 1892, I returned from Russia to England. I was tired by the time I got there, and ran straight into a string of things I didn't particularly want to do. A friend asked me to recommend a place for her to live. I hate to be asked to make recommendations of this sort. My brother was at home, an invalid, and I did my best to nurse him. Finally I decided I just had to get some rest, so I rented a room in Sussex Gardens, one of those places where all the paying guests come down to join in a communal meal at dinner time.

I had hardly been in my new room for forty-eight hours before I discovered my landlady considered herself a medium. I didn't mind that, as mediumship is a gift to be treasured, but what irritated me was that she was a constant talker: jabber, jabber, jabber. And I was the perfect target, as she had heard of my reputation in the psychic field, and she could talk to me about such things without being thought a lunatic.

One night she called to me, "Come into the parlour. The ghost of my late husband, Henry, is here." I came down to take a look but frankly I could not see Henry. The house cat did though. Tabby stared into the corner with eyes as big as saucers, tail straight and fur bristling.

My little room was invaded at all hours by my too interested landlady, who would suddenly remember some thrilling psychic experience she wanted to share with me. At length I took to my bed for three days, not in the least ill, but simply for a much needed rest in the midst of these excitements.

A day or two after emerging from this haven of peace, I received a visit from a young lady whose parents were well known to me in Yorkshire, and who had recently become engaged to a very rich man, many years her senior, in fact, considerably older than her own father, who had lately passed away. The daughters of this family were all devoted to their father, and most of the visit was occupied in giving me details of his last illness, and in my sympathizing with her. It was, in fact, far more a visit of condolence than of congratulations upon her future prospects of happiness. As to the latter, I found it difficult to be quite truthful.

To marry a man old enough to be your grandfather struck me as risky, even with all the advantages that wealth can bring to life.

The young woman in question did not at all resent my frankness, but assured me that her greatest consolation in thinking of her late father was the fact that she was about to make a marriage which he had hoped for. On his deathbed she had told him she had decided upon it. "He was so happy about it", she said simply.

Then I received a note from a younger sister of the coming bride, and was given an invitation to a large musical party. It was within a stone's throw of Sussex Gardens, and I came down to dinner at 7.30p.m., intending to dress later and go to the party at around nine.

For an hour or so before dinner, I had been conscious of a growing despondency to which I could attribute no cause, and it increased so much during dinner that Mrs. Peters, my landlady, asked me if I was ill.

"No – not unwell – but for some reason absolutely miserable, and I cannot imagine why."

"Then you have not heard bad news?" was the next remark. "I feared you must have done so, seeing you so silent and not eating."

In answer I mumbled that I had not even the excuse of hearing other peoples' misfortunes, for a young lady had called on me, who was about to make what the world calls a very successful marriage. I did not, however, mention her name as Mrs. Peters knew none of my acquaintances.

Dinner over, I felt still so unaccountably wretched that I determined to give up the musical party. Mrs. Peters did her best to defeat this decision but, finding me determined, she then said, "Well, if you have quite determined not to go, let's go ourselves and hold a little seance together to see what the spirits have to say about it."

Even though Mrs. Peters annoyed me by invading my privacy, I knew she was quite good at mediumship, so I accepted the suggestion.

I wrote a brief note declining the party, and joined my landlady in her room.

We sat in the dark for some moments, and then I heard a swish from Mrs. Peters' silk gown, and knew she was tracing out words with her hand in a fashion of her own.

"It is a spirit that your young lady friend brought with her," she announced at length. "The spirit has remained with *you*, and is depressed and worried about this marriage you spoke of. She wants you to try and break it off. She seems to have been related to this lady during her life on earth, perhaps a godmother. Anyway, she takes a great interest in her."

"Will she give a name?" I asked.

"Eliza is all I get," Mrs. Peters replied.

"Eliza," I searched my memory. Yes, I did recall that my young friend had been given that nickname by a relative.

I asked if a surname could be given, thinking it would be Waverley – the family name, but Mrs. Peters said definitely it was not Waverley. I found later that Aunt Eliza (after whom the girl had been nicknamed) had a different last name.

The message that came through at our informal seance, however, did not induce me to take the responsibility to break off any marriage. I had neither the authority nor the influence to make any such attempt.

Sunday came and with it came the bride's younger sister to see me. She joined the group at the dinner table. Looking at her, I saw that she was staring at Mrs. Peters who, in turn, was intently staring back at her. Our hostess seemed to become uneasy, closed her eyes and seemed almost to be asleep.

I shook her back to alertness.

The young girl apologised for her staring, saying, "I am so sorry that my staring at you made you feel ill."

"No, my dear... it was not your staring that entranced me. *It was that man standing over you.* He had his hands on your shoulders, and was trying hard to influence you while you resisted, and the whole conflict of both wills was thrown upon me. That is why I *passed out* to avoid the mental pressure," she gasped out.

"Could you describe the man?" I asked.

"Very clearly," she said. "I identify him as the father of the woman who plans to become a bride. Waverley is the name. Does that have meaning?"

"Yes, it does definitely," I responded. "Can you find out what message he has for his daughter?"

"No! No, Miss Bates! Don't ask me to do that! Dear Henry never liked my taking messages from strangers. I promised him that I would never do it without his permission. It upsets me so much, and I feel so weak already."

The young sister and I left, promising to come back later and see if we could do anything for her.

The young sister was very interested after hearing the medium recite the name of her father. In fact, she was anxious to pay Mrs. Peters a second visit.

I knocked on Mrs. Peters' door. She called out "Come in". I found her standing, and in a state of excitement. She had, in fact, been on the point of coming to us when I entered.

"Dear Henry told me to take that message after all," were the words with which she greeted me. "There was some misunderstanding between the father and this daughter, and he wants her to know that it is all right now." (This seemed most improbable to me, as I knew that the devoted daughter and father were always on terms of harmony. *Yet it proved to be quite true.*)

Mrs. Peters continued : "He is very much upset about this marriage. He tells me he was so anxious for it when on this side, but now he sees all the difficulties and possible dangers. He says it is too late to stop the marriage now, but that it is extremely important that his daughter get all financial interests secure before she marries. The settlement must be legally documented, otherwise she will lose all her deserved inheritance when her old husband comes over, which is not too distant in time." The medium went on, "He is most concerned about this because he says it was he who urged the marriage upon her."

I spent the next half hour as a sort of messenger between Mrs. Peters in her room, and the bride's sister in mine. Needless to say, I personally knew nothing of these legal aspects.

Mrs. Peters, on the contrary, seemed to know everything connected with the estate and the marriage settlement: *except the fact that such had not yet been signed.* Why this special limitation in the father's knowledge, it is impossible to say. He certainly showed no limitation in his knowledge of the bridegroom's character and disposition, and gave detailed instructions as to how his daughter could most successfully relate to the old man.

My advice to the young sister was to say nothing of the subject to her older sister but she, wisely as it turned out, determined to take the responsibility of telling her *everything.* She telegraphed me next day, asking if she and her sister might come for further spirit information from Mrs. Peters.

This was done, and they arrived, with several photographs of both the father and the prospective bridegroom for identification. The younger of the two tried a little trick on Mrs. Peters by saying that the picture of the father was the bridegroom, and the bridegroom was the father. But Mrs. Peters would have none of it. She immediately reversed the pictures, and acclaimed the one of the real father correctly. "This is the face I saw," she stated with decision.

Mrs. Peters may have been a "jabberer", as I have mentioned, but as a medium that lady was no fake. I came really to appreciate her.

The bride-to-be requested a private interview with Mrs. Peters. Of course, I knew nothing of this interview, nor would I feel at liberty to speak of it if I did. It was strictly private between the two women. I may, though, be permitted to say that I have the bride's own assurance that the accurate knowledge given her about how to deal with and love her future husband made a world of difference to the happiness of her married life to the old gentleman.

During that interview Mrs. Peters also told her the length of time she would be married before the death of her husband, and the prophesy was accurately fulfilled.

I am happy to add that the marriage turned out a complete success, and that a marriage settlement was made in accordance with the father's wishes, although neither trustees nor principal in the transaction had any idea that the actual arrangements were in any way due to the strongly expressed wishes of a discarnate spirit.

I have frequently heard it expressed by some people, that psychic gifts should not be used for such mundane things as financial arrangements. I have always stated that this is *nonsense* – financial affairs are very much part of life on this side of the veil, and can be dealt with on the level of intelligence.

Often I find myself thinking: if discarnate spirits *don't* trouble about the personal affairs of those on earth, the "cui bono" argument is hurled at them. If they *do*, they are called irreverent! It's the old cliché of "The Old Man and the Donkey".

I don't recall whether or not I mentioned that the Waverley family had been friends of my family for years. Occasionally I had visited them. I am reminded of another psychic incident which took place when I was staying in their house in the country, a year or two earlier than the marriage prophesy. I have reserved it purposely as a sequel to that story, although this is not in its proper chronological order.

In the year 1889, I was spending a pleasant fortnight with the Waverleys in Yorkshire, at the very time when a dear old friend of mine (Mrs. Tennant) was dying in London.

I had seen my friend only a week or two before, but had no knowledge of her illness, as we were not in touch too often, although there was a strong bond of affection between us.

I did not even hear of her death in fact until a few weeks after it took place, having missed the obituary in the newspapers. Mrs. Tennant's sister, Mrs. Lane, wrote to tell me the details. I had left Yorkshire, and was staying with cousins in Worcestershire. Thinking over the dates mentioned in describing the illness, I realized with pained surprise that she had died at the time when I was enjoying a party in Yorkshire, given by the Waverleys.

It seemed terrible to think that such a loved friend should have died without my being even aware of it. Me – who has always regarded herself as being much attuned to psychic impressions. Then, suddenly, I remembered a curious little incident connected with that party.

I had been admiring a pretty little grey kitten that was sleeping on a pillow by the hearth. After the gentlemen joined us, I went into conversation with my host when I noticed a small *black* kitten run past my dress. Probably I should have remarked upon it had we been less occupied in talking, for I am very fond of cats. I did glance up, as a matter of fact, and satisfied myself that it was not the little grey coloured kitty which was still sleeping on the pillow. This kitten was definitely *black* and not grey.

I thought no more about it until the guests had left and Mrs. Waverley and I were going upstairs to bed. These friends well knew of my interest in spiritualism and, while not much into it themselves, they would occasionally make comments. On this occasion she said, rather mysteriously, *"I think something will happen to you tonight."*

I laughed it, off thinking she was trying to pull my leg, as it were. But Mrs. Waverley was quite in earnest. She said to me, "While you were talking to my husband, I saw a black kitten run across your dress – just opposite me."

"Well, of course I saw the kitten!" I answered, to her surprise, "But there is nothing very remarkable about a black kitten in the house."

"But we have no black kitten in the house, or anywhere on the premises. Where did it go? You never saw it again? No, it somehow did not strike me as being an ordinary kitten, and I did not imagine that anyone, till that moment, had seen it but myself."

It was a fact that no one but Mrs. Waverley and I had seen any kitten but the grey one, which was a pet in the house.

Thinking this over in the light of the sad news of my dear old friend's death, and noting the correspondence in the time of her death and the appearance of the mysterious black kitten – it was impossible not to ask in the depths of my heart whether, perchance, the spirit of my faithful friend of long standing had been trying to send me some symbol of her passing.

I think that my dear "friend mother", as she called herself, would have explained this manifestation very simply: she had had a black cat as a pet for many years. In time it died, and she buried it in her yard. That pet was very dear to her... so sending that symbol to me at the time of her death was most appropriate.

I will finish this session of haunting experiences on a merrier note, by telling an amusing episode connected with the evening of the black kitten's appearance.

Among the guests invited to the Waverleys' party was a clergyman. A "squarson" is the name for such a gentleman in Yorkshire, which means, I believe, a squire who is a parson.

This particular specimen of the genus was both a vegetarian and a celibate. This latter fact I had heard expressed in the neighbourhood, that he had remained a bachelor owing to religious scruples. The vegetarianism was equally certain, as he was most particular that none of his dishes at meals contained any meat. No poultry or fish either.

When the gentlemen had joined us in the drawing room, the conversation turned upon psychic matters, as it often seems to do when I'm around. I was asked to recount some of my materialization seance experiences while I was in America a few years before. This clergyman denounced them all.

Although he believed that everything might have happened as described, he was equally certain that the whole thing was the work of the devil. Perhaps it is best to mention that he did not use that exact expression.

Religious conversations have a way of becoming an argument, so our host tried to come to the rescue by jokingly saying, "That red chap with the horns and pointed tail, certainly does get blamed for a lot of things!"

Instead of laughing, the parson took it seriously, and straight out said that my spirit investigations were in direct opposition to the Bible – quoting: "*We are specially warned in the Scriptures that: "...In the latter days, seducing spirits shall arise, and will deceive the elect".*"

He glared at me, as he said this.

At this fatal moment, when theological doctrine was descending on my unhappy head, a really brilliant thought occurred to me.

Was it a seducing spirit or a friendly intelligence who came to my rescue, and reminded me that my opponent had only quoted half the text – *the half that suited him.*

I pointed this out.

"What do you mean?" he asked, puzzled.
So I finished the other half of the text for him: *"In the latter days seducing spirits shall arise, forbidding to marry and commanding to abstain from meats."*

There was dead silence, and the argument stopped right there. If I had been a celibate and vegetarian, it was not a text I should have chosen to clinch my argument!

....

CLINICAL REPORT

End of Session Eight. With the last remark, "...forbidding to marry and commanding to abstain from meats," client just stopped speaking and aroused herself from hypnosis without any instruction from me, entirely of her own volition. When I enquired as to what had aroused her she said she had no idea. I explained that I had not given her any instruction to do so. Her only explanation was that perhaps Katharine had completed enough of the story for one day. As previously my client had total amnesia regarding the content of the session and was very happy with the outcome.

For my personal comments on this session, see over ...

PERSONAL NOTATIONS TO MYSELF:

It becomes obvious to my clinical observation that, with each session, Sarah Channing and Katharine Bates become increasingly integrated in personality. In other words, client is subconsciously coming to recognize that her experiences as Katharine Bates, in her past lifetime, and Sarah Channing, in her current lifetime, are actually a continuum of the same individual (possibly I should say "spirit") telling of experiences that happened to her in diverse time and space relationships under diverse name identification.

Psychologically, it is interesting to observe that an integration of personality is happening, rather than a disassociation of personality. This is demonstrated by the method of her arousal from this session.

As I have noted, client seems to enjoy each session and eagerly looks forward to listening to the tapes of each session. Above all she looks forward to subsequent sessions with great relish.

Session Nine arranged.

Chapter Nine

LADY CAITHNESS OF AVENUE WAGRAM

Pre-session interview. Carried out the usual checks and everything appeared normal. A little time was spent talking about the previous session and the mode of her awakening at the end. Sarah was unable to add any further observations as to the cause and was happy to believe that it was Katharine who made the decision.

Almost to confirm my previous notes concerning integration of personalities the client has frequently referred to Katharine as me on several occasions during the course of this interview.

Sarah had obviously thought the incident Katharine had had with the "squarson" highly amusing for every time it was mentioned she burst out laughing. It is said that laughter is the best medicine for many ills. No doubt Sarah built up a store of good medicine as a result of this. Again we spent about twenty minutes talking generally about the subjects of spiritualism and reincarnation.

I eventually curtailed the conversation as I feared little time would be left for the regression itself. Immediately on relaxing on the couch Sarah slipped into her usual deep trance and on the arranged signal recommenced her story as Katharine.

Session 9

Having spent the winter months of 1894 (from January to April) in Egypt, I was returning to England. My route was via Paris, and I was hopeful of meeting the famous Countess Caithness, to whom I had a letter of introduction. Lady Caithness had her exclusive mansion on Avenue Wagram in Paris, and was internationally recognized as an authority on occultism. She had written a book on Black Magic and, quite honestly, there were those who thought it would be safer if she were locked up in an asylum, as it was said she imagined herself a reincarnation of Mary, Queen of Scots, who was beheaded.

As for myself, I was without prejudice and, after meeting her, decided she was both charming and had her head "well screwed on", as the saying goes. I saw her daily for a week, and never once heard her mention thinking of herself as Mary Queen of Scots although I confess I did see half a dozen portraits of the unfortunate Queen displayed on various walls of her home.

It can truthfully be stated that she did have claim to a close relationship with Mary Queen of Scots. I do not know really what her views were on the matter. I had heard Lord Monkswell speak on the theory of reincarnation, his ideas being that one short earth life gave small scope for the evolution of the soul, and that a repeating of lifetime after lifetime was needed by the inner (real) SELF to reach the peak in its development, so as to be able to advance to ever higher realms of consciousness. He had further interesting ideas that it might be quite possible for the same spirit to manifest in two bodies simultaneously and that, say, the judge and the criminal might conceivably be one and the same individual in two personalities. Lord Monkswell was an interesting man.

It is possible that Lady Caithness held similar views. If so, her personality was certainly a case in point, although she never expressed any such opinion to me.

The Countess's home was like a miniature palace, and was evidently used as a school of occult instruction. When I arrived, I was conducted to a large parlour in which were a dozen or so courtly ladies and one man, whom they surrounded. He was a priest: Abbé Petit. He was a short, stout man with a bald head. He reminded me of Friar Tuck, of Robin Hood fame. Fat as he was, he held the group of women in awed fascination. These female worshippers, surrounding the little priest, were hanging on every word the man spoke, as he discoursed on understanding old truths through modern concepts. It reminded me of a scene in Molière's *Les Femmes Savantes.*

To tell the truth, there was a certain humour about the whole situation and I had trouble not giggling, but my dignity did not allow that. Fortunately, Countess Caithness entered about then, and a hush came over the room. She was magnificently gowned in flowing white satin, and a priceless tiara adorned with jewels encircled her head. That she was queen in her castle there was no doubt.

Lady Caithness came directly up to me. "Katharine Bates, I had notice of your coming. Your reputation as a psychic investigator, with an especial interest in spiritualism, has preceded you. Pray, come and sit beside me while M. l'Abbé reads his paper explaining how he can no longer blind his eyes to the new age of science that is dawning, but that he sincerely remains a loyal son of the Church, if the Church will allow him to do so."

M. l'Abbé concluded his talk to the women by announcing that a special seance was to be held exclusively in the presence of Lady Caithness and two female mediums, but that they would be notified when a seance open to them was permitted. The group of fawning women was dismissed.

Lady Caithness went on, "I am sorry that I cannot invite you to this seance tomorrow night, but that is to be devoted entirely to receiving last instructions for the completion of M. l'Abbé's paper, the beginning of which you heard tonight. Later in the week we will hold a special seance in your honour."

Never once did this wonderful woman try to patronize me; I was accepted on an equal level.

"Of course," I responded, and hastened to assure Lady Caithness of my full understanding. "I will await word from you."

"I shall notify you. You will be with us again, so I will not say goodbye."

I left the house on Avenue Wagram, wondering what the future would hold.

A full day passed with no notice. Also, the morning of the next, a long morning which I spent at the Louvre. I arrived at my hotel around 1.30p.m. but there was no letter in my box. I wondered if my invitation had been put out of mind. I was wrong. An hour later, a *dépêche* letter arrived for me.

Lady Caithness wrote *to beg pardon for the delay in communication, and asked if I would make a point of being with her that evening. A private seance had been arranged just for me.*

That evening I arrived at the mansion shortly before nine, and was conducted into her private quarters. The room in which I found myself was lavishly furnished but, to me, the most striking thing in the room was a full-length, life-sized painting of Mary herself, so arranged that a hidden lamp threw its soft light on the delicate features of the Queen, while hanging velvet curtains of deep crimson on either side concealed the frame of the picture. An illusion was conveyed that a living woman was standing there, ready to receive her guests.

I have never seen anything more perfect than the way in which this impression was conveyed.

Lady Caithness and Abbé Petit entered together and, after greetings, conducted me to the seance room. Two French woman mediums were already in the room – one older and one younger. I was told that they were mother and daughter. Frankly, I was not too impressed, as there was something coarse about them. Noting my reaction, Lady Caithness whispered to me, "Be not surprised: often, mediumship is found among the peasant people. They are excellent physical mediums when working together." They must have been so, unless one supposes that Lady Caithness and the Abbé Petit were wrong in their judgement. That was not likely.

We sat down at a large wooden table, polished, but without covering of any kind, and having only one solid support to it, a single central pillar, spreading out in the usual fashion at the base. I had noticed this table when first entering the room.

Resting on top of the table was a printed alphabet card and a long pencil pointer.

At a side table, placed some distance away, I saw an attractive young French lady, to whom I had not been introduced. She was giving her full attention to the "automatic writing" which seemed to be flowing out of her. She was the secretary of the Countess, I believe. This young lady had no possible connection with the table.

The light in the room was lowered, but was still sufficient for full visibility. The seance began with a few words of prayer from the Abbé, asking for strength, guidance and protection.

The process was as follows:

First the Countess, and then I, took the printed alphabet and pointed silently and at a fair pace to the letters: going on from one to the other without pause. At the letter needed, the table did not rise but gave a sound more like a bang that a rap. I had never heard anything *quite* so loud and definite in my long investigation. The sound seemed to come from *within the wood*, as in expected spirit rapping when these are genuine, but it was far louder and more rapid than the usual seance rap. There was no hesitation, no gathering up of force. Any amount of vitality was evidently present and the intelligence, from whatever source, was unerring. The Countess and I were the only two persons who held the alphabet and pointer and when *she* held it, the mediums could not have seen the letters from their position at the table with regard to hers. Yet the letters were *banged* out (I can use no other expression) with absolute accuracy, and at a pace which, quick to start with, became more and more rapid, as we wearied of the monotonous task and handed the alphabet to each other in turn.

When these loud bangs came, I could trace the reverberation in the wood, and it seemed to me practically impossible that the old and young French mediums could be producing them by deceptive methods, while sitting clearly visible to us with immovable faces, the daughter writing down the letters as quickly as these were indicated.

One does not feel quite comfortable about making investigations in a private house, at a seance in which one is the guest of honour. However, a psychic investigator does have a responsibility to detect trickery, if such is present.

If the women were tricking, and I caught them at it, there was always a chance of a disagreeable scene with people of their class.

On the other hand, it was losing an opportunity to refrain as a mere matter of courtesy. Also, I comforted myself by thinking that, if anyone needed to feel ashamed, it would be the ones who cheated and not the detective.

So I pushed my chair a little nearer to the table and, the next time the Countess took the alphabet from me and the bangs were in full swing, I moved my foot around the pillar forming the central leg of the table. Nothing. There was no sign of any deception there, yet I could positively and distinctly hear the reverberation of the loud bang on the wood between me and the centre of the table, while my foot was exploring beneath the table. One thought did occur to me, which was that possibly the pillar leg was hollow, and a rod might be extended up through a hole in the floor, up the hollow leg to bang against the under surface of the table's top. But this idea was destroyed when the table began to tip and glide, and when I felt the heavy table seem to float beneath our hands.

The letters written down so rapidly by the young medium at first seemed a jumble but, when the sitting was over, the Abbé and I were able to make out the words and sentences without much difficulty. Mostly it seemed to be a sort of spiritual message, probably more directed towards the priest than anyone else in the room. It was interesting, but the only sentences which remain in my memory are these two: "Christianity is a stretching down of the Divinity of Man," and "Theosophy is the attempt of Man, by his own interpretation, to reach the Divine."

These sentences struck me as being both terse and true.

We sat at the seance from 9.30p.m. till 1.00a.m. I was getting tired, and it was a relief when Lady Caithness suggested we adjourn and have a snack.

After some social conversation I said "Good night."

On the following day, I was invited to lunch with Lady Caithness at 2.00p.m. and, being a punctual person, I arrived at that hour. The doorman announced that his mistress had not yet emerged from her bedroom, and showed me into the parlour, where I awaited her. Shortly, I was joined there by the Abbé, who politely expressed his sorrow that he had not known of my earlier arrival. Then the Countess joined us, and the three of us developed a growing friendship.

The day following that most enjoyable luncheon, I announced that I had to go on my way. I left with a happy remembrance of her and her hospitality to me during my stay in Paris. She made me promise to let her know whenever I might happen to be passing through France. I wrote to her the next year, when about to make a short stay in Paris on returning from Algeria, and received an answer from the Riviera. She had been wintering there. She begged me to go to the Avenue Wagram when I arrived, and find out the latest news of her.

Ten days later I *did* go to her house "palace", and was interviewed by a lady secretary (not the one I had seen before). She was not at all courteous, and gave me the impression that she quickly disposed of persons who claimed acquaintance with the Countess. So I handed her my card, and prepared to leave. The moment she saw my name her manner entirely changed, and became as servile as it had previously been "cavalier".

"Miss Katharine Bates? I see. I shall communicate at once with her ladyship. I had no idea you were Miss Bates. Pray excuse me: so many come and ask for the Countess, and we have to be very particular. But, of course, *you* must be the lady that Lady Caithness is so very fond of. She has mentioned you often, and asked that we extend to you every consideration."

And that is my last recollection of the magnificent woman, who died a few months later. No, not absolutely my last recollection: I had heard her body had been taken to Scotland, at her request, to be buried near Mary Queen of Scots. I made it a point to find her grave.

The plain stone slab and simple inscription seemed at first a curious contrast to the gorgeous manner in which she lived. Yet I am inclined to think that they represented a side of her character which was quite as real as the side of pomp.

In like manner, no one who knew of her only as a "wild visionary" could have realized that the shrewd, practical woman of business was she who shared the personality of the Countess of Caithness and the Duchesse de Pomar.

I remember that Mr. Frederic Myers made the same remark to me after a visit he paid to her, just following my return to England, for the purpose of arranging matters with regard to her generous bequest to the British Society for Psychic Research.

M. l'Abbé, I never saw again.

....

CLINICAL REPORT

End of Session Nine. Very little to report about in this session. Sarah behaved in her normal way but this time I aroused her from trance, and again she had no conscious memory of what had occurred in the session.

For those not well versed in the subject of hypnotic induction it is worth noting that the couch itself had by now become an automatic signal for Sarah to let go of the conscious world and enter her subconscious world through the medium of trance. This phenomenon is often referred to as kinesthetic anchoring. In other words the actual physical act of getting on the couch and lying down on it itself acts as a trigger for the client to re-enter trance.

The clever hypnotist uses this naturally occurring phenomenon in order to save time and effort in having to re-induce trance in his subject. He does this by giving the client a post-hypnotic suggestion that on the next occasion they come for therapy when they lie down on the couch or sit in a certain chair or hear a special word they will immediately enter trance. My students often ask how or why this happens. Whilst there are long and quite complex medical and psychological descriptions of what occurs, I prefer to keep things simple so I tell my students that we are after all creatures of habit and the power of pre-supposition is truly awesome.

There is a definite continuity in our work together.

PERSONAL NOTATION TO MYSELF:

Sarah Channing, in telling of her life as Katharine Bates, is reciting in an almost impersonal way. She does not seem to get emotionally involved in what she is reciting. Her experience is much as a person would have in telling a blind person what is being seen on a television screen.

Session Ten has been arranged.

Chapter Ten

MY DEVELOPING MEDIUMSHIP

Pre-session interview. Carried out the usual checks and again spent some time discussing the tape from the previous session. Sarah was particularly interested in finding out how much of the attributes of a person's past life were carried forward into the next. Her search for knowledge was not so much about herself and Katharine Bates but more about Mary Queen of Scots and Lady Caithness. She was interested in the common connections which existed between the two. Both were of noble birth, both were Scottish, etc. She did however, say that she had already discovered a number of connections between herself as Sarah and as Katharine but seemed a little reticent to discuss them further.

As usual Sarah slipped into trance as soon as she was on the couch and recommenced her story as Katharine.

Session 10

From Paris to England is not far, and my next reminiscence is connected with the University of Oxford. It was while there that I had my first personal experience with trance mediumship. Trance Mediumship is where a sensitive enters a sort of relaxed reverie state (called trance) in which the mind is opened to impressions coming through from the other side. The experience is much like holding an intimate conversation inside your head, in which a spirit presents a communication. Here is how it came about:

I was spending a few days there with a friend in the spring of 1896, and went with her one afternoon to an Oxford tea party, with its usual mixture of married and unmarried women, a few professors and more than a few undergraduates.

Among the latter, I chanced to hear the name of a Church of England bishop whom I had first met and known rather intimately when we had been much younger. Also, I had known rather well the woman he had married in those far-off days, so my curiosity was aroused to know if the young man at this Oxford party should, by any chance, be their son.

I introduced myself, and found that my surmise was correct. We were soon engaged in an interesting conversation about his parents, especially his mother who had died when he had been barely three years old. He knew little or nothing about her. His father had married again, and his grandmother (still alive in 1896) had never cared for the woman who had been his mother – from feelings of jealousy, probably – so there was no one for the young man to ask about her. He was delighted to hear my girlish recollections of her.

"Do come and have tea with me tomorrow afternoon," he said eagerly. "I have a few old photographs taken of my mother when she was young, and I would like to know which of them you consider the best."

Of course, I agreed to go. We met and discussed the photographs. I selected the one I thought was best.

Returning home from my visit with him that February evening, I was conscious of an unaccountable depression and a certain amount of nervous irritability, which other sensitives will understand, and which often precedes a psychic happening. Just after I had finished my dinner, it struck me suddenly, and *for the first time*, that my discomfort might be connected with my afternoon visit. It occurred to me that this young man's mother might be striving to impress her presence upon me in some way! It was as though her spirit desired communication with me.

Mentally I responded, and I promised my willingness to listen to anything she might wish to say.

Having given this promise, all disturbing influences disappeared. I told the friend with whom I was staying about this mental spirit visitation.

Next morning after breakfast, my hostess said practically, "Now, do get this matter off your mind at once, or you will be worried about it all day. I will be tending to some work in other parts of the house, so you can have this room entirely to yourself."

I sat down quietly, alone. I closed my eyes, and opened myself to whatever might come in from the other side.

A very beautiful message was given to me by the friend of my girlhood.

She was evidently much concerned about something connected with her son, whom I had met at the Oxford tea-party. Of what this could be, I was in complete ignorance. His mother – now in spirit – seemed anxious not to betray confidences, so her words which came through to me – in my trance state – were very guarded. As the impressions came through, there was evidently nothing in the least dishonourable or in any way *unworthy* about her son. Rather, I gathered, that he might be contemplating some step which she, from her wider outlook, considered undesirable and inexpedient, possibly even disastrous in the future.

It was no business of mine, and I make it a point not to "try to guess" more than I am told, and to forget what I *am* told where the affairs of other people are involved.

This is easy for me to do as a rule, but in this case one sentence remains in my memory from the son's mother. These were her last beautiful words in a loving message:

"Tell my darling boy that life is so solemn, and true love so sacred a thing. Tell him to be very sure, lest he lose the substance in pursuing the shadow."

The message gave me a problem to solve: what should I do with it?

In the first place, Mr. Blake-Mason might resent my writing to him in such a sentimental vein, especially since he had no knowledge of psychic matters. Second, he might mistakenly suppose that I had been probing into his private business, to give him a personal warning, under cover of his deceased mother's wishes. Third, he might consider me a lunatic, giving him such a message. Fourth, it might convey the impression that his mother had some secret access to his most private affairs, and was advising him from the unseen world, in which case, he might get too wrapped up in psychic matters, to the exclusion of his daily activities. In my personal observations this is not an uncommon happening among young people – not to mention other possibilities of psychic disaster for inexperienced investigators.

It required careful consideration on my part, as to what was best to do Finally, I decided it was best to send the message to him, and trust the consequences to a Higher Wisdom.

I did this, adding a few words of explanation and also warning him not to become too much involved in psychic matters. Unfortunately, I added that *there was no need for him to respond to this letter.*

I left Oxford the next day, and true to my suggestion that there was no need for a response to my letter, there was none. So I was much in the dark as to just what his reaction to my letter might be. It was not until four years later that I found out.

I put the matter more or less out of my head.

As mentioned, it was some four years before the corroboration of that message came to me. It came in a curious way.

A cousin of mine, having been wounded in the South Africa War or Boer War as it has become known, was sent to a London hospital for treatment. It was a rather serious wound, so he was confined to the hospital for several weeks during the London season of 1899. During that time I paid him an occasional visit. On one of my visits, he happened to mention the name of a ward nurse, commenting how capable and kind she was. Then he added, "She is the daughter of the Bishop of Granchester. You know almost everybody, Cousin Katie! Perhaps you know her?" he said, smiling.

I responded, a bit surprised, "No, I don't know her, but I knew her mother and father very well, many years ago."

Nothing would satisfy him but that I should meet her before I left the hospital. I promised to do so.

I asked at the hospital's reception desk if I might see her, when she might be free? They buzzed her room. In a few moments she came out, and we went together into a quiet lounge. She was a pretty girl somewhere in her late twenties. I introduced myself. When she learned my name she exclaimed, "You are Katharine Bates! My goodness, yes! I have heard of you! My brother, Frank, told me all about meeting you at Oxford."

We chatted together for a full half hour. As I was leaving, I asked one last question, "Did your brother ever tell you of a letter he received from me in Oxford"

"Oh yes," she answered without a touch of embarrassment.

Then I continued, "I never heard from him about it. I told him there was no need to write at the time, but I have always wondered how he might have taken the message I had received from the spirit of his mother?"

"Did Frank never write?" she asked in astonishment. "I know he intended to. That message was of great importance to him, and *I have the best of reasons for knowing that that message from his mother, which you told him of, made a tremendous difference in his life.*"

I thanked her, and left without further comment. As I have said, it was no affair of mine, from first to last; but the verification, after such a lapse of time, was an elation to me in verifying the accuracy of my trance mediumship.

Another shake of the kaleidoscope.

I found myself at Wimbledon, staying with a friend (now passed onwards) who had a house not far from the Common, and with whom I often spent a few days when in London.

On this occasion, she had asked some friends to meet me at tea, amongst them Mr. Alfred Wedgwood, to whom I had introduced her some years previously, along with his wife and my friends Mr. V. C. Desertis and his wife. It was a pleasant reunion as the couples were there for this afternoon social occasion.

A Miss Farquhar, whom I knew very slightly, was sharing a sofa with me, she sitting at one end and I at the other, leaving a vacant space between us. Mrs. Wedgwood was talking to Mr. Desertis at that moment when suddenly he looked across the room at our sofa, and began describing – in detail – an old man sitting between Miss Farquhar and myself, leaning on a cane and wearing a soft felt hat.

"He has long, grey hair almost down to his coat collar. He is a very kindly-looking old man."

Mrs. Wedgwood, staring at the vacant space between us, added, "I see him too. His hair is more than grey: it is white."

"And curly and long?"

"Yes, curly and quite long, reaching to his collar," Mrs. Desertis spoke up.

Then Mr. Desertis said of the phantom, whom the others seemed to be seeing, "Then it cannot possibly be my father as his hair, while white, was quite short."

Bur Mrs. Wedgwood still insisted that she had never seen such a visitation more distinctly, whether we recognized him or not.

What was particularly interesting to me was that I found myself spontaneously slipping into the trance mediumship skill which I had found myself developing previously. I began to see the phantom form of the old man too. Mediumship seems to be something which occurs at unexpected times to those sensitive to experiencing manifestations of the unseen world. I seemed to have a natural talent in that direction, which increasingly developed.

I should here mention that I had been sleeping very poorly in my friend's house for some past nights. I regretted this, as I planned to visit another friend shortly, in Windsor, and wanted to be bright for coming festivities. However, these bad nights later proved to have some connection with the apparition of the benevolent old gentleman just described.

Now I will continue the sequence of events.

The manifestation of the spirit of the old gentleman was more or less relegated to the position of a memory, as other interesting matters arose in conversation.

The following day, Miss Farquhar wrote a note to my hostess asking if she might come to tea towards the end of the week as she had something interesting to tell us.

In due course, when at tea, she gave us a more detailed description of the old gentleman. She continued, "In fact, I have felt his presence so strongly, I determined to try and find out something about him.

"I went to an elderly lady I knew, one of the oldest inhabitants of the area, and asked if she knew anything about the previous inhabitants of this house. She told me an elderly couple had lived here, that the husband had died and that, although the wife lived away from Wimbledon now, she could not bear to part with the house which her late husband had been so fond of. So she decided to let it. It would seem that she is the present landlady."

This was true, said my hostess. The house had been let through an agent, and the present owner lived in a distant county. Other than that, nothing was known of her personally by my friend.

Miss Farquhar continued, "Hearing that the old man was so devoted to the house suggested a reason for Mrs. Wedgwood's seeing his spirit here, so I asked the old lady to describe the late husband. She did so, *and her description was word for word exactly as I had seen his spirit visitation.* Also, she added that he was somewhat of an invalid, often sat indoors with a hat on for fear of draughts and carried a cane upon which he constantly leaned for support."

We applauded Miss Farquhar's detective instincts, and promised to let Mrs. Wedgwood know about the matter. Mrs. Wedgwood took it all as factual, only remarking that she felt that someone should find out more about the old man.

A sudden thought struck me that my disturbed nights, in a very cheerful bedroom, might possibly be connected with the same old man. I asked Mrs. Wedgwood to come up into my room before she returned to London, and I told her of my difficulty in sleeping: in fact, that I had not had a peaceful night since I arrived. "Can you find out the cause?" I asked her.

Mrs. Wedgwood replied immediately, "There is not the slightest doubt of the cause. It is that old man, of course. He is earthbound, I expect, and is haunting the house. If you can, you had better take a message from him. That will help him go on into the light, which illuminates the doorway to the unseen world. I would help you if I could, but I shall be late for my return to London if I do not start at once."

Next morning, I relaxed into the reverie of mediumship, opened my awareness and his message came through while I was in trance.

He said pathetically:

"You must forgive me for disturbing you so much, I was so anxious to convey a message to my wife, and I recognized you were a sensitive and could take it from me. That lady had called me earth-bound but, if I am, it is only through my deep love for my dear wife, and I am permitted to watch over her. I was drawn here by my old affection for this house, and also by your presence here, knowing you could help me."

He then gave the message, of which I can only say that it was most touching in its expression of deep affection and watchful care for his widow. He departed my presence adding, "Now that this is conveyed, when it is possible, pass it on to her and tell her I am well and fine on this side, and look forward to her joining me. Shortly now it will be. You will sleep well in this room from now on."

He was right. From that time forward during my visit, I have seldom enjoyed more perfect sleep.

I told this message to my hostess. As we did not know this lady's present address, my hostess and I settled that she would lock up the message, in the hope that someday we might be able to forward it.

A year later I had the most unpleasant experience of becoming seriously ill. A clairvoyant medium assured me that this resulted from the message remaining undelivered, and the old man's consciousness's frantic endeavours to reach his wife's consciousness, assuring her he was well and fine. I told my Wimbledon friend that something *must* be done. She must make every effort to procure the lady's address, and send on the spirit message from her beloved husband.

Under pressure of this determination, the address was finally located, and the message sent on to the wife.

Yet a still further unpleasant experience was to follow.

I wrote a courteous letter to the old lady, enclosing the message. I expressed my sincere regrets at the delay in its delivery, and hoped that she would excuse my tardiness in sending it over more than a year after the message originally came through my mediumship. I further expressed the hope that his message of love and devotion to her would bring her much happiness.

To my almost shocked surprise, her reply to my letter was filled with wrath.

The wife to whom the message was sent was furious. She had no belief in such spirit nonsense. She added, "My dear husband was the perfect gentleman, and he was not old – not a day over sixty-eight when he died."

It would have been amusing if it had not been rather pitiful to think of a perfect gentleman as a "young" man of sixty-eight, trying so hard to reach such a vindictive, hard-headed fanatic.

Later, I heard from my hostess who had sent on my letter containing the message, that she, also, had received a letter back, asking whether or not I was a lunatic.

One has to be philosophical about such things, I suppose, as to how some in our *seen* world fail to "welcome" a communication from the *unseen* world. Sadly, this is far too often the case. The marvel to me is that LOVE can still be stronger than DEATH, in the face of such ingratitude and stupidity!

As my mediumship advanced, so did my extreme sensitiveness advance in perceiving the atmosphere of psychic rooms, especially rooms in which one sleeps. I will tell you of such an incident.

I was paying a first visit to a new friend whom I had met. She lived in the south of England, and a very bright, cheerful room had been allotted to me there.

From the very first night, I felt a strong influence of a man in the room. Note, I do not say the influence of a *strong* man; on the contrary, the character appeared to me that of an essentially weak man – weak rather than wicked, however, very sensual, self-indulgent and greatly lacking in grit and will-power.

My current hostess had two sons, one whom I knew and the other whom I had never met. The influence was certainly not that of the son I knew, as he was a fine soldier and "hard as nails", as men would say.

I feared it might be the other son however, and took an early opportunity of asking to see a photograph of the latter. My mind was quite set at rest. It was certainly not this man's influence that I felt so strongly in my room.

Asking my hostess *who* had chiefly occupied the room, she said at once, "Both my sons have slept there at different times. What seems to be the matter with the room?"

I told her, "Now that I am quite convinced that neither of your sons is implicated, I will describe the character of a man whom I feel sure must have slept in that room, and has left a strong psychic influence behind him."

I then mentioned the characteristics I have described.

My hostess was amazed. She said nothing at that moment, but crossed the room to a cabinet and brought out a photograph of a man whom I had never seen, and placed it in my hands.

"I am bound to confess," she added, "you have exactly described the character of my brother-in-law, who certainly has occupied the room more than once."

The sequel to this incident is rather significant.

A couple of years later this lady and I, having succumbed to influenza, were both recovering in the same room in the same hospital. During our mutual recovery, she gave me the piece of news that her brother-in-law had died from a very painful disease. "At any rate, he wrote me a very touching letter when I lost a very dear relation, wondering why such a valuable life should have been taken, and such a "useless dog" as himself be left alive."

I further learned that this poor man had only just passed over when I had slept in that room those two years before. It came to my mind that, beyond doubt, his spirit had left his body in a very bewildered and perplexed state of being. With my advancing sensitivity, I now realized why I had felt his presence so clearly: partly from having sensed his character so strongly and partly from the hope he obviously held that I might be able to help him on his new plane of life.

Now that I had been given the full details of the case, my attitude changed completely, and I sent a prayer to help him. Personally, I have never had any difficulty in realizing the power of prayer for those who have passed beyond our mortal sight.

Surely we are one large family, whether here or there? The best way to make children love each other is to persuade them to *help* each other. It seems to be a rule that applies to the entire universe, not just the tiny portion of it that we know.

Anyway, I am quite sure in this case that my prayers did help and comfort this poor man in his dark experience.

In a dream he came to me, and thanked me for my compassion. Then he left, and he has never come back again.

Beyond question some will say, "Could not someone else have done the work equally well – possibly an administering angel in the other realm?"

The answer is, "Certainly equally well, and probably far better."

But the point is that it happened to be a bit of work put into *my* hands, and I did my best. What more can any of us say?

I can say, "Thank God for the gift of my developing mediumship which has come my way."

....

CLINICAL REPORT

End of Session Ten. There is really little I need to comment on in reporting on this session. It pretty well tells its own story. Suffice it to say that the client aroused from hypnosis pleasantly, as usual. She had amnesia as to what she had recited, upon returning from trance. However, in listening to the recording of the session, she commented that she did have flashes of conscious recall, as it went along.

Session Eleven arranged.

Chapter Eleven

A MEDIUMISTIC LOOK AT HAUNTINGS

Pre-session Interview. Carried our usual checks with client and had a general discussion of the content of the last session. Much of our discussion was concerned with how our minds are able to store information about past lives seemingly at a subconscious level whilst this information is normally not available to us in consciousness. I offered her various theories about this curious subject but eventually the client said that she wished to keep an open mind as she felt Katharine may have something to say on the matter. Again there was no differentiation between Sarah and Katharine. The client is clearly integrating the psyche of both personalities with no apparent problems or discomfort.

Session 11

England has always been renowned for hauntings. Reports of haunted castles and manors and mysterious apparitions are prevalent in the British countryside. Here are two incidents (one a dead ghost haunting, and the other a live ghost haunting) which occurred to me only shortly after those I told of in our previous session. These hauntings took place in the same year of 1896.

I was staying in London during the season, and some girlfriends were anxious for me to meet a woman who was well-known in society. Her name was Mrs. Halifax, and she was quite pompous. As so often happens under forced circumstances, we were not in the least interested in each other, but that has nothing to do with my haunting story.

My girlfriends had arranged the meeting, and they begged me to come in good time, as Mrs. Halifax had several other engagements, and could not remain with us for long.

So, I dressed hurriedly in order to keep the appointment and went to the house feeling (I must admit) rather bored by the whole arrangement, little dreaming it would provide such a unique mediumistic experience for me.

Mrs. Halifax turned out to be a very wealthy woman, yet very uninteresting from my point of view. Very likely I was equally uninteresting to her, as I mentioned. I knew she had a son and daughter with her, but I did not know that another young man (whose *face* I had not seen) was also a son of hers. I talked to the mother for about a quarter of an hour, and then turned with relief to the other son whom she had mentioned, and with whom I found I had several mutual acquaintances. We had a pleasant chat.

Meanwhile, some other guests had arrived. Amongst these I noticed the entrance of a man whom I instinctively did not like. He looked dissipated and conceited. I did not speak to this man, but my strong impression about him is a factor in my story.

When Mrs. Halifax rose to take her leave, followed by her son and daughter, I noticed the second young man, whose face I had not seen, rise to leave also. I had not seen his face for the very good reason that he had been sitting behind me.

I did not see his face even now. My attention had been diverted from the Halifax party as they rose to leave, and I only noticed the *back* of the second young man as they left the room. I was told later that he was the other son of Mrs. Halifax.

As my mediumship developed, I often tried to help sad or wandering spirits by praying for them, when made conscious of their presence near me, in the same way as I had done in the brother-in-law case which I have already told you about.

When I awoke that night, following the meeting with Mrs. Halifax and her family, and felt a presence near me, it did not alarm me at first in any way.

When I was fully aroused however, I immediately realized that this was no poor bewildered spirit, but that it was very malignant and revengeful: *I did not recognize the sex at that moment.* In fact, it came to my consciousness that right now my prayers were needed by no spirit more urgently than my own.

I could sense it keenly. There was something dangerous in the room – something or someone far too actively wrathful to listen to any prayer.

This conviction grew so strong upon me that I lit a candle and, getting out of bed, prayed for protection against the evil thing that was present in my room.

I think I must have remained at least ten minutes on my knees, and I can remember distinctly the feeling of alarm and hopelessness that came over me. How little my prayers *seemed* to avail.

Shortly however I felt the evil presence leave, and I returned to my bed feeling quite calm and strong, and fell asleep pleasantly.

As a developing medium, I have always found it as easy to communicate with incarnate spirits at a distance as with discarnate ones so, on awakening in the morning, remembering my disagreeable experience, I asked a friend at breakfast what was the meaning of it.

I had made up my mind that if it were in any way connected with the visitors of the previous afternoon, it must be the dissipated man I had taken an aversion to.

To my surprise I was told it was not that person, but was the younger Halifax son. "It was Henry Halifax. It is a spirit which has been haunting him, and it came to you afterwards."

Now, I had not even seen the face of this young man, as I mentioned, and I could not think of any fanciful accusation against him. "Are you sure it was Henry Halifax?" I asked.

"Yes! It was Henry Halifax."

"But I did not even see him," I argued.

"True: but you were sitting with your back to him all afternoon. Surely you must know that the back is more psychicly sensitive than any other part of the body?"

I said nothing, and nothing further was said about the malignant spirit beyond the fact that it was haunting Henry Halifax.

That morning I went down to my Wimbledon friend for a night. I arrived in time for luncheon on Saturday morning and, after a walk on the Common in the afternoon, my friend suggested going to a certain florist's shop, as she wanted to buy some flowers for her drawing room.

I had previously met the florist's wife. She struck me as a rather "weird" sort of person, who had been introduced to me by Mr. Myers of the Society for Psychic Research. However, once I got to know her better, she did not seem so weird and, really, she had had some wonderful psychic experiences, as had her children. These had been carefully documented by the Society.

Mrs. Levret was the name of the florist's wife and, when our flower purchasing business was completed, she turned to me and said, "Katharine Bates, I am glad to see you again. Have you had any interesting psychic experiences since we met last?"

Now although Mrs. Levret was very psychic and had had many curious experiences of her own she was the kind of person who kept rather quiet about herself, and I had never known her before to express an interest in anyone else.

It flashed through my mind to tell her of my disagreeable experience in the bedroom. I told her of the evil presence I had sensed, which had finally left when I prayed.

From my words, she must have gathered that I supposed the haunting spirit to be that of a *man*.

As we left the flower shop, my hostess said pleasantly, "We must hurry home now Mrs. Levret, but do come up tomorrow and see Miss Bates. She does not leave until that evening, and you ladies can have a nice talk together."

Mrs. Levret promised to come, and appeared next morning. She came straight up to my bedroom and we had an interesting talk about her own strange adventures.

Suddenly she looked up and said, "How about the young man? What are you going to do about him?"

"What young man?" I asked, puzzled. "What can I do about which young man?"

The Halifax incident had so completely faded from my mind that I could not for the moment recall what she meant.

"The young man you told me about yesterday after-noon," Mrs. Levret answered.

"But I can't do anything about him. What *should* I do?"

Mrs. Levret continued:

"I have been thinking a good deal about that young man since yesterday. It seemed to take a sort of hold upon me. It comes to my sensing *that it is a young woman who is haunting him – a young woman who is not in his own rank in life – someone whom he wronged.*"

I was astounded by these words, and still more by the keen interest Mrs. Levret showed in the subject.

"But what can I do in the matter?" was my next question.

"They give me to understand that the young man must be made to confess. He will never have any peace until he does. It seems you are the only one who might get him to confess."

Now there could be no question of confession in the seen world, as the young man was a perfect stranger to me, and there was little chance of our ever meeting again. But I was aware that Mrs. Levret was not speaking of the other plane, so I agreed to take pencil and paper, and see if I could bring the spirit of Henry Halifax to me and, having done so, whether I could induce him to tell the truth.

His spirit responded to my plea. Thus to me he came, but for a long while would say neither "Yes" nor "No". *"What business is it of yours?"* was his constant reply to my questions. I am bound to admit that the spirit of the man was right – from the ordinary point of view.

Truly it *was* no business of mine, but Mrs. Levret was in earnest and had impressed me so strongly that I felt I must persevere, in the young man's own interests.

So I explained I had no wish to pry into his private affairs from unworthy curiosity but that I had, myself, felt the malignant presence that was said to be haunting him and, being told that only confession would remove it, I hoped he would consider the matter seriously before obstinately closing the door of opportunity for freedom from the haunting spirit.

A long pause. I felt the angry mood was passing over, and when my hand was next automatically influenced to write, there was an apology for his stubborn reception of my efforts to help him.

A confession came forth.

He told me that he had betrayed a young woman of a different rank of life from his own. She had died in childbirth the *preceding summer*, and had died cursing him. He confessed that, ever since, he had been haunted by her presence – a consciousness of a malignant spirit tempting him to his own destruction. The agony was so great he did not think he could bear it and had almost decided to put an end to his life (little realizing that, bad as this life might be, the next phase would be far worse for him).

After trying to soothe him without in any way minimizing the weight of his sin or attempting to lessen his remorse for it, it struck me I should make an attempt to communicate with the spirit of the defiled girl who had died. I dropped myself into a trance, and mentally asked for *her* spirit to come – to try to influence her in the direction of forgiveness.

The poor young woman had trusted him and had been deceived. Literally she had almost been raped into motherhood. Little wonder she haunted the man who had wronged her so terribly, through pure selfishness, and any love she had ever felt for him had since turned to deadly hate!

Her spirit came to me while I was deep in trance mediumship. At first, she was completely vindictive but, by degrees, a more womanly view of the subject seemed to come to her. After all, he was the father of her child, the poor little baby that had, mercifully, followed its mother into the unseen world. She had loved him once. I made the most of this point. Grudgingly, she gave a promise to cease at least this revengeful haunting, even though she could not entirely release the hate towards the one who had wronged her so deeply.

Having obtained this promise, I let her go. Mrs. Levret smiled at me, and also took her leave.

I have given this account of haunting by a vengeful spirit at length, as it may be helpful to others dealing with vengeful spirits. Also because, on my return to London, *every point of this case was corroborated.*

Truthfully, it took time and tact before the case was completed.

First, I learned that Henry Halifax was not welcomed in his home any longer, and had only come when the other children had prevailed upon his mother to allow him. They did not know the true facts of the case. They only knew he was moody, unhappy and discontented.

Now, I happened to know another friend of the Halifax family; a woman considerably older than the young people mentioned; and she had some knowledge and respect for psychic possibilities. I determined to lay the whole story before her, trusting her honour to keep it confidential, and not to allow prejudice against Henry Halifax to arise in her mind.

She promised.

She had known the family from her childhood, and through her I discovered that the confession of Henry Halifax – to the spirit of the wronged girl – was no illusion on my part, *but the absolute truth.*

As he was young, handsome and rich, with all the world before him (he was only twenty-four at the time) the lady had been greatly puzzled by his intense depression, and told me he was constantly speaking of suicide. His parents had supposed it was a nervous breakdown. She had the good fortune to know an intimate man friend of his: a man with whom she shared confidences. He told her of the situation, and that the young woman, of lower social position, had died in childbirth the previous summer.

How great was her astonishment to find the whole story had been made known to me through spirit connections. First, my experiencing of the malignant spirit. Second, my going to Wimbledon next day, and the circumstances of meeting the wife of the florist, Mrs. Levret. Third, Mrs. Levret's quite accurate psychic impressions of the case. Fourth, my two interviews, first with the betrayer and then with the betrayed on the psychic plane, which ended in a confession and a promise to end the haunting.

I have never seen Henry Halifax again, but I trust the confession was as efficacious as Mrs. Levret was told it would be. I did learn, however, that the gentleman in question is now happily married and therefore presumably no longer haunted by the vengeful spirit who has long since, it is my deepest trust, found peace in a higher world than his.

As I am telling of my mediumistic experiences with hauntings, I had another that same year. In its way, this was just the opposite of the Henry Halifax case which was a haunting by the so-called dead, while the one I will tell now is a haunting by the so-called living. It happened while I was staying in Cambridge for the first time in my life.

Oxford I have known since girlhood, but this was my first visit to the sister University of Cambridge although I have of course met many men who graduated from there. Not knowing the town of Cambridge myself, I had never made it a subject of discussion and was not even aware that such a street as Trumpington existed in that city.

In any case, the fact is that I did *not* know that a very dear friend of mine, who later in life became a judge, had ever lived in this street. He became a sailor as a young man and went up to Cambridge University comparatively late. This was shortly before my acquaintance with him began.

My not knowing Cambridge at all, the question of where he lived there had never come up. I rather took it for granted that he was living on the college campus (Peterhouse). We developed a warm friendship, but when he began to get amorous I had to break it off. Looking back on it now, maybe I made the mistake of my life in being such a prude. This all happened more than a quarter of a century ago. I had heard he had made a success in the legal profession, but that was all I knew about him.

After staying for a week with friends in the neighbourhood of Cambridge in 1896, I moved into the city and took rooms there for a month. During that time, I invited one of these friends to stay with me, as a guest.

I came upon these special rooms in a curious way. I went searching to find suitable lodging, but nothing seemed quite right. By the merest chance, I heard that possibly I might find what I wanted in an historic house in Trumpington Street. I went there, only to find the rooms, while vacant, were not ready for immediate occupancy, as friends of the owner were coming to stay for a few days.

"But I want them for a *month*," I exclaimed.

The landlady was firm; she could not disappoint her friends, to whom she had promised their use.

While I was disappointed, I did admire her honour in keeping her promise to her friends. So I decided to look at the rooms while I was there, just in case they might be available in the future.

We went upstairs. The rooms were exactly what I wanted, so it ended by my agreeing to take them a week later.

It was in this casual way that I entered the house about the middle of May 1896. My friend was not able to join me until the morning after my arrival, so I spent the first evening alone and retired early. I slept well during the earlier part of the night, but awoke around 2.00a.m. having dreamed of the very Cambridge man I previously mentioned who had not been in my thoughts for many years.

Even when fully awake, I somehow still felt the presence of this man in the room with me. I fell asleep again, and there he was once more in my dream, chiding me for not allowing ourselves to have enjoyed an *affaire* in the past. He even suggested that things might have been better for both of us had we married. He even scolded me a little.

This sort of thing went on for the rest of the night. Either I woke up with a start, still feeling his presence in the room, or I sank into a troubled sleep, to be once more at the mercy of his reproaches!

When morning came I was thankful to get up, and when my friend arrived at about noon and asked me how I had slept in the newly rented rooms, I told her that my night had been troubled by dreams of an "almost" boyfriend of whom she had never heard.

"Oh well, we all dream about would-be loves sometimes," she said, "but I'm afraid in this case your dreams were not pleasant; you look tired out!"

We joked about the matter a little, and then let it drop.

But the following night the troubled dream was renewed. Even then I did not connect it with the room in which I was sleeping, so I said nothing on the subject to my friend the next day.

But on the *third* night, matters had gone beyond a joke. The man's influence in the room was stronger than ever, and his reproaches more accusing. Added to this was my exasperation at having had three mostly sleepless nights.

However, instead of feeling depressed, I had the good sense to express myself to this male influence as though the man himself were listening to me.

I spoke forcefully, "I have no unkind feelings towards you. In fact, I once almost loved you. However, if you have nothing better to do than to come to me nightly and keep me awake, it just proves I was right in not marrying you! You have nothing whatever to do with my life now! SO GO!"

Standing up in this way to the "ghostly influence" somehow made me feel much better, so I crawled into bed and had an excellent, dreamless sleep.

My sensitiveness to understanding things of this nature suggested to me that this past man friend *must have some special connection with the house.* In the morning, I confessed frankly to my invited guest that the presence (I did not use the term ghost to her) was haunting the place. I told her, "I am going to find out if he ever had rooms here."

As things turned out it was easier for me to make that decision than to solve the mystery. His college career in Cambridge had been some twenty five years past. When I questioned the young daughter of the landlady as to how long her parents had lived in the house, she said at once, "Just seventeen years, Ma'am. Father and Mother came here the year I was born."

This did not help me much. I asked who had rented the house previously. She referred the question to her mother, who told me it had been taken from some people who had left Cambridge. *"God alone knows where they are now."*

This was a cul-de-sac for me. However, I determined to go on with my investigations. Definitely, I felt that my repeated sleepless nights' experiences *must* have some foundation in fact.

The woman saw I was not satisfied. "Did you especially want to know about anyone who lived here long ago?" she ventured.

"Yes. I wanted to find out whether an old friend of mine ever lived in this house. He belonged to the Peterhouse fraternity," was my answer.

"Ah, then I am sure he would not have lodged here," said the present owner confidently. "None of the Peterhouse gentlemen come here. It is always the Pembroke men who come to this house."

That was as far as I got. It seemed fated that I would hear no more about my living ghost.

A few days later though, things took a turn.

I was told quite casually that Mr. Pound, the well-known Cambridge postmaster, had occupied the house years before. He was regarded as quite the historian of Cambridge.

One day I went into the post office to buy some stamps and Mr. Pound himself handed them to me. Here was my chance to get some further information. I must admit I was a little timid about asking, as it was hardly likely he would remember the names of all undergraduates in the University who might have lodged with him some twenty five years back. However, I took the chance and asked him, "Is it true, Mr. Pound, that you lived many years ago at the old rooming house in Trumpington Street?"

"Quite true," was the ready answer. "I went there in '55."

I continued to ask, "By any chance, do you recall a gentleman who may have lived there a good deal later, about '70 I would think. Forbes was the name."

Mr. Pound looked up with a beaming smile. "Mr. Forbes," he said, "why of course, I remember him well. In fact, we roomed together for better than a year, while we were going to college." Then, telling his assistant to take over the stamp window, he took me into his parlour and brought forth a large photograph album. There was my early friend, sure enough, with his big dog – the very photograph he had given me in the early days of our acquaintance.

Mr. Pound was full of reminiscences. My friend seemed to have been a close friend of his, and it was some moments before I could squeeze in my critical question. It seemed almost impossible to expect him to remember the exact room which had been occupied by Mr. Forbes, considering that there were several sets of rooms in the old house.

But he remembered it well. "Which room he slept in, you ask? Why of course, I remember it distinctly. He had the large front sitting room with the bedroom at the back of it."

Correct! So I was indeed living and sleeping in the very rooms he had occupied in that house for over a year. My intuitive impression had proved correct. My feeling of his "living ghost" in my room had been confirmed.

I thanked the postmaster and, before I left, he added, "As far as I know he is still living although for the life of me I couldn't tell you where."

I later related this incident to Mr. Myers of the Psychic Research Society. Both he and Professor Sidgwick were very interested in the case, as they explained that there were fifty accounts of hauntings by the dead, in England, to one such example of haunting by the living.

To me, the salient fact remains that, after a lapse of nearly thirty years, I traced the rooms occupied by an old acquaintance (who definitely had romantic notions about me) in a city I had never before visited, and that this knowledge did not come to me by chance, *but as the result of a series of my personal investigations in a house and in a room of which I had had absolutely no previous knowledge.*

In retrospect I have asked myself many times since, *"Do you suppose the spirit of Mr. Forbes came to me, in my dreams, while I was half asleep (you might call it entranced)?"* *If so, I definitely feel that he was conscious of my presence too.*

As I reflect on it now, maybe I should have married the man. A gentleman who still holds a flame in his heart for a woman thus strongly so as to manifest his invisible presence to her after almost thirty years is really quite a gentleman!

Of course, I am happy just as I am but it is certainly not impossible that I would have been even happier as the wife of Mr. Forbes.

....

CLINICAL REPORT

End of Session Eleven. As usual, client roused from hypnosis pleasantly. Session interspersed with long silences. However it was clear from the client's facial expressions during these silences that she was experiencing something, but despite my prompting she declined to verbalize her thoughts. She had no exact memory as to what she had recalled. There was a smile on her face, and she didn't know just why. But I did!

Session Twelve was arranged.

Chapter Twelve

BACK TO THE USA

Pre-session Interview. Carried out usual checks with client and discussed the content of the tape from the previous session. Client said she had found some of the content disturbing because it brought back some painful memories in this life. We spent a little while discussing how these could be dealt with, with me now clearly in the role of psychotherapist rather than as an explorer of the paranormal. Clearly Sarah has been repressing these memories and at some stage will need to free herself from the power that they hold over her.

Before I could pursue the subject further my client slowly got up from her chair, walked over to the couch, lay down and instantly entered trance. In order to oblige her I whispered the words, and Sarah returned to her story of Katharine.

I need to return to these repressed memories later.

Session 12

I made my second visit to America in the year of the Diamond Jubilee, 1897. My purpose was to meet the internationally famous spirit medium, Mrs. Piper, and to secure some sittings with her. I was writing some articles for *Borderland* at the time, and the editor asked me personally to interview the renowned American sensitive. This proved no easy task.

My visit to Boston unfortunately occurred at the very time when an organized attempt was being made by the American branch of the Society for Psychic Research to obtain evidence of communication with the late Stainton Moses, through his "controls".

In vain I wrote to Dr. Hodgson (to whom I carried letters of introduction) telling him of my chief reason for visiting the USA a second time. Even the plea that I had known Mr. Stainton Moses in earth life, and that we had several intimate friends in common, was of no avail.

Dr. Hodgson wrote back, expressing regrets, but assured me that *no* sitting could be allowed under existing circumstances, and that it was impossible to make any exceptions to this rule.

I seemed to have run into another of those cul-de-sacs that ever and anon haunt my life.

Then a bright idea struck me:

Why not ask the UNSEEN themselves for a decision in the matter.

I wrote again to Dr. Hodgson, suggesting this idea, and mentioning that I would arrive in Boston on a certain date, and that I would be staying at the *Hotel Bellevue* in that city.

Following my arrival and settling in, and quite early in the morning, Dr. Hodgson came to call on me.

It was my first meeting with this famous man. What a totally delightful personality he was. At the very moment of our meeting he spoke right out and, with a half-rueful amusement at his own discomfiture, said: "Well, you've got to come! They insist upon it, so there is nothing more to be said!"

Any preconceived ideas of a critical, elderly, white-haired professor, taking himself very seriously, were instantly dispersed on my meeting Dr. Hodgson, and this was the beginning of a sincere and loyal friendship between us which lasted for nine years on this plane and will last, I trust and believe, through whatever forms of existence may succeed to this one.

Dr. Hodgson and I made arrangements for us to meet next morning at Arlington Heights, where my first sitting with Mrs. Piper took place, and where I met for the first time this refined and interesting woman.

I was told that, with the advent of Stainton Moses' controls, the character of Mrs. Piper's mediumship had undergone a complete change. The former communications through voice ceased and gave place to automatic writing, except at the moment of return to the physical body, when a chance sentence or two might be articulated during the transition period, but these were not always intelligible to the listener.

Entering trance, Mrs. Piper's arm and hand became "dead" and limp, as unconsciousness set in; the blood departed, leaving them as white as that of a corpse. By degrees the dead look disappeared, blood flowed again through the veins, and the hand groped towards the pencil held out by Dr. Hodgson, and finally grasped it.

Dr. Hodgson's long experience and patience were invaluable in deciphering almost illegible script. The encouragement he gave to all attempts at definite communications, the care with which he repeated again and again a question not fully comprehended – all this, combined with intelligent criticism, alert dispassionate judgement and balance of mind, made him one of the world's master investigators of psychic phenomena.

The first thing that struck me in the two sittings I had with Mrs. Piper was the complete breakdown of the Thought Transference Theory as accounting for her automatic writing.

It became obvious that the reason for the request for my presence at Arlington Heights was to facilitate Mr. Stainton Moses' spirit communication, as I had known him in earth life.

Again and again I asked for names of friends we had mutually known, but the results were negative.

Yet, next day, some of these names would appear spontaneously in the script.

References were made to Mr. Moses' appreciation of music, including an inquiry asking if Mrs. Stratton still played BACH. Also, reference came through referring to his visiting the Strattons, and finding them playing duets together, in London.

These things seemed superficial at the time, but later showed proof of the genuineness of the phenomena. Mrs. Stratton confirmed that Mr. Moses liked music, but she denied that she and her husband had played duets in his presence. Mr. Stratton, however, corrected this impression, and reminded her of several occasions when Mr. Moses came to see them at the University, and found them at the piano and had requested they should finish the passage or movement.

These slight but evidential incidents, forgotten by Mrs. Stratton herself, and unknown to me, were conveyed quite correctly in the automatic writing through Mrs. Piper – three thousand miles across the Atlantic – and nearly six years after the death of Mr. Stainton Moses.

To me, the most convincing test of all that came through was the mention of a Mrs. Lane – the lady to whom Mr. Moses had been engaged when he had passed onwards. This was very convincing as very few of his friends, even in England had known of this engagement. Dr. Hodgson had never met Stainton Moses in earth life, and had no knowledge of it. It was only by chance that I knew anything of the matter, through once meeting the lady.

During my second sitting with Mrs. Piper, I mentioned meeting this lady, and the "control" at once asked if I had met a *sister* also.

I answered, "No."

The writing at once continued, "She *has* a sister, who has been the cause of deep sorrow in her life. You will find this is true when you return to England."

Subsequently I found this to be absolutely true: however, it took some investigation on my part to unearth the truth. On my return to England, when I saw her next, I asked Mrs. Stratton about any sister. She said, "I have come to know Mrs. Lane very well and, as far as I know, there is no sister. I am sure she would have told me if a sister had caused her sorrow, as you mention."

I persevered however in searching out the truth of the matter by writing to Mrs. Lane herself (an entire stranger to me) and asked if she would care to hear the references to herself in the Piper seance, and if so, would she come and lunch with me?

She came, and when I reached the passage about the sister, expecting that she would endorse Mrs. Stratton's denial, to my great surprise her eyes filled with tears.

The tears ran down her cheeks, and she said in a sobbing voice, "That is the most convincing proof of his communication to me from spirit, as I have never mentioned my sister to anyone, other than my dearest Stainton. She was the cause of the greatest sorrow in my life: a confidence only myself and my beloved shared."

At the second sitting with Mrs. Piper, the spirit of Mr. Stainton Moses spoke of a valuable watch he owned and expressed regret that it had not been given to Mrs. Lane at the time of his death.

I knew nothing about any watch of his, but on checking with the executors of his estate later on it was reported that there had been such a watch, of considerable value. Upon the death of Mr. Moses it had been given (with the approval of Mrs. Lane) to the son of an esteemed friend.

This executor also told me, as a curious coincidence, that when he had been visiting with friends in Sussex Gardens, he and his wife had been given a similar message purporting to come from Stainton Moses.

Another incident regarding this watch occurred, which I remember well. Mr. and Mrs. Harrington had come to tea with me one afternoon. As part of our conversation, Mrs. Harrington remarked that she had heard mention of Mr. Moses' watch through a medium. It was of research interest to me hearing mention of the watch while in Sussex Gardens, London, and later in Arlington Heights, Boston.

During the Arlington Heights sitting (the second one I had with Mrs. Piper) Mr. Moses' spirit also referred to an important manuscript which he had hidden in his home. Following the directions given, the document was found.

After my sittings with Mrs. Piper, my next psychic happening, on my return visit to America, was in connection with a Mr. Knapton Thompson, a New York businessman who had invented a new kind of smokeless stove. It must have been a good invention, as several of these stoves had been put in public buildings, including the Smithsonian Institute in Washington, D.C.

Mr. Thompson had a sincere interest in psychic phenomena, and had become interested in the New York medium, Mrs. Stoddard Gray. He had found her a competent medium, and had written to tell Mr. Stead of his experiences.

Mr. Stead turned this gentleman over to me, with a request that I should see the man, and give a report on the spirit experiences he had claimed to have witnessed.

With an introduction through Mr. Stead, I asked Mr. Thompson to call upon me and arranged to be present at the next holding of Mrs. Stoddard Gray's circle. He said he was satisfied that her mediumship was genuine. As will be recalled, I concurred: excellent mediumship.

Accordingly, I went with Mr. Thompson to a Gray's seance with every expectation of an excellent sitting. My expectations were entirely destroyed however, owing to the presence of a vulgar man who made inane remarks, cracked sordid jokes and antagonized every respectable person attending the seance. Results were negative.

The afternoon was spoilt for all there, and I remarked upon this to a pleasant young American lady, who had been seated beside me.

"Indeed yes; he was exasperating!" she said, completely understanding.

She was obviously a person of high quality, so I asked how she had happened to be attending the seance.

She explained her position readily, and it was very interesting to me.

She had been invited to attend Mrs. Gray's seances several weeks previously by a cousin who thought the experience might be amusing.

"We came at first just for a joke," she said, "but phenomena happened which interested me so much that I went again several times and, until today, each of her seances had been fruitful.

Then she told me of her first sitting with the medium.

I had noticed she was wearing a very beautiful scarab ring. It was exquisite. I commented on it. "Yes, it is a Tiffany setting," she observed, seeing my eyes drawn to it. She took off the ring, and handed it to me.

"That ring is really the cause of my being here today," she continued. "It was given to me by a famous American egyptologist, who had been a friend of my father for years. He made a pet of me when I was a child, and I begged him for it. When I was going to be married last year he insisted on having it set for me by Tiffany as a wedding present and then he told me that it was a genuine *Cleopatra* relic, taken from an Egyptian tomb.

"To cut a long story short," she went on, "in that first seance which I attended with my cousin, I had worn the ring but it was concealed beneath my gloves. I did not take them off until the seance room was darkened, so no one knew of it. In the dark, I took off my gloves when I found we were to sit in a circle holding hands. One of the first materializations announced that it was to be the ancient Egyptian Queen, Cleopatra.

"The Cleopatra form had no sooner materialised in the room than it dashed directly towards me in the darkness, seized my right hand, amongst all the hands in a circle of twenty people or more, almost tore this special ring from my finger and said, in a tone of indescribable longing: "Mine! Mine! Ah, *Chem! Chem!*"."

This was startling in the extreme, and was amplified further by the repeated mentioning of Chem, which is the ancient name for Egypt.

This incident had sufficiently impressed her that she had attended several of Mrs. Gray's seances prior to our meeting.

During this, my second visit to America, I had the good fortune to gain the friendship of Margaret Whiting, the acclaimed authoress. We were together often in Boston and, during one of our conversations at her *Brunswick Hotel* suite, she told me of the visit of Lady Henry Somerset and Miss Frances Willard to that city some five years previously. Miss Whiting also mentioned a friend who had accompanied these two ladies, who had died suddenly in the Boston Hospital.

"I never met this party," said Margaret Whiting, "but they were shocked to hear of her sudden and quite unexpected death. I am not sure of this, but I have heard that she has become the "Julia" spirit control in Mr. Stead's spiritualistic investigations."

The day following the fiasco seance just described, Mr. Knapton Thompson called at my hotel to invite me to attend another seance being presented under the mediumship of Mrs. Stoddard Gray. I accepted the invitation, very much hoping that things would go much more smoothly this time. It was announced as a "writing seance" that afternoon.

As was usual, Mrs. Gray's son was the active assistant. On this occasion, he had an alphabet mounted on a large card. His job was to point to the various letters in turn, as they were spiritually indicated, while his mother wrote them down. By this process, various messages were secured.

A sizeable group had gathered and when my turn came to receive a message, thinking I would attempt to verify Margaret Whiting's story if possible, my first question was, "Can Stead's Julia give me her surname?"

"Julia O." was spelt out, and then the "O" was given again.

"They often do that," said Mrs. Gray casually, "begin the name over again, I mean."

The rest of the letters indicated corroborated the surname mentioned by Miss Whiting.

Then I asked, "In what country did you pass onward?"

"*America*," was spelt out at once.

"In what city?"

"*Boston.*"

"In what kind of residence did you die?"

"*In a hospital,*" was again spelt out.

"How long ago?"

"*Five years,*" was the answer.

I must note here that Miss Whiting had *not* mentioned the number of years; only having said, "A few years ago," when speaking of the sudden death of the friend in the hospital. *Five years* was true.

My last question was, "What was your age when you made the transition?"

"*Twenty-three,*" was the answer.

This last, I felt must be wrong. Margaret Whiting had not mentioned any age, but it seemed to me unlikely that so young a woman would have been travelling around the country with two older woman lecturers.

When these answers were being given, Mrs. Gray's son asked if he might place his hand on my wrist to balance the magnetic energies.

I was acquainted with the "muscle reading" method of the renowned Washington Irving Bishop in demonstrating "mind reading". I said that it would be agreeable, but that I was going to keep my eyes closed, so my muscles would not give him any unconscious indications.

When I sent these answers to Mr. Stead on returning to England, I wrote down Julia O (ignoring the repetition of the O) and, in connection with the other answers, told him of my previous conversation with Miss Whiting, which reduced the whole episode to one of possible Thought Transference.

In answering me he said, "I am glad Julia was able to give her name, even if it was Thought Transference, but, as a matter of fact, it was not her whole name which you received – she always signed her letters to me 'Julia O.O..'." This makes a good bit of evidence for the spiritualistic genuineness of the phenomenon, seeing that the second O *had* been given, but discarded by Mrs. Gray and myself as a repetition of the first letter of the *surname*.

To resume my experiences in America with Mr. Thompson, who was my frequent escort while I was in New York, he and I attended later another public seance given by Mrs. Gray. Mr Thompson was sitting on one side of me.

After some "materializations" for other members of the circle had appeared, Mrs. Gray announced that Stead's 'Julia' was present in the cabinet and wished to speak to me.

I promptly went up to the cabinet, and the form came out and stood, quite evident, even in the dim light of the room. It was a female form, and she seized my hands with every appearance of delight, and her grasp was firm. I have an artistic sense of always noticing hands. They always seem to me to indicate the character of a person very closely, and I am attracted by people who have graceful hands, and I tend to reject people with clumsy, ugly fingers.

Now, I had noted that the medium's hands were broad, short and flabby. The hands which grasped mine now were, on the contrary, small, narrow and graceful – very feminine hands.

Mr. Thompson had come up beside me to greet "Julia", and I whispered to him, "Ask Julia if there was not a mistake about her age this afternoon."

"No. You ask the question yourself, Miss Bates," he answered.

So I said rather eagerly, "Julia tell us, please, if there was not a mistake as to your age when you passed over – the answer was twenty-three. Is that correct?"

The spirit body of the lovely woman emphatically shook its head, signifying "no" as the reply to the last question, but no sounds came from her lips.

She made a little gesture of rather helpless dissent, and Mrs. Gray, who stood by, explained that most likely all her strength had gone to building up the materialized body sufficiently to make it visible to us. Julia bowed her head in assent to this and then, still speechless, retired once more behind the cabinet curtains.

I did not mention this appearance of Julia when I next wrote to Mr. Stead on my return, as I wanted to see what his own comments might be, as a test of the genuineness of the phenomenon, but he said nothing about it in his return letter. So I let the matter go.

Mr. Stead and I had always been good correspondents, so a week later I wrote him another letter, and put a casual P.S. to it.

In answering my letter, he replied – also in a P.S:

"In answering your query – yes, Julia told me she had appeared to you in New York, *but that she could not give you her age on that occasion, because she was not accustomed to speaking through the embodiment.*"

Now, in sending the list of questions and answers to Mr. Stead, I merely marked against the answer as to her age, "twenty-three," – but I had never hinted to him that I had asked her to correctly state her age of passing while in New York, or that she had been unable to speak on that occasion.

Again, this stood as pretty sound objective evidence of the genuineness of Julia's spirit manifestation.

I will now give an accounting of Mr. Knapton Thompson's spirit interview with his daughter who had passed onwards some years previously. This occurred on the same evening, at the same seance when Julia appeared to me.

On this special evening, his daughter materialized and came forth from the cabinet. As Mr. Thompson was sitting next to me, I could distinctly hear Mrs. Gray whisper to him, "Would you like to take your daughter into the other room, Mr. Thompson? It is rather crowded here tonight. You will find it quieter in there."

Mr. Thompson got up at once, greeted the materialized form, and they disappeared through the folding door to the adjoining room. In giving my attention to other matters as the seance unfolded, I had quite forgotten the absence of Mr. Thompson, until I found that he had returned to his seat beside me. I asked him quietly where his daughter was. He answered equally quietly, "She did not dare to come back into this crowded room so, after our half hour chat, she dematerialized in the other room, and I returned alone."

Imagination? Fanciful wishing? Not likely in a hardheaded New York businessman and successful inventor. He was certainly under the impression that he could be trusted to recognize his own daughter when allowed the privilege of half-an-hour's conversation with her in a private room.

I will end this narration of my psychic experiences while on my second trip to the USA by presenting a case of a rare form of clairvoyant projection perception which occurred to me personally. It concerns a man whom I was never privileged to meet in the same world but with whom I must have had some soul connection in the unseen: Dr. Nikola

Tesla, the electrical genius. This report, while lacking any physical ground of proof or mental ground of comprehension, holds great importance to my life.

I had hoped to have had the opportunity of meeting this acclaimed man during my last stay in Philadelphia, in March of 1897, but was disappointed in this expectation. It was an unfulfilled wish during this lifetime.

At the time of my first visit to America, back in 1885, I had not the faintest conception of Tesla's work or what he was on the track of discovering. All I knew about him was through some rumours that had trickled over to England, that he was either a visionary, a madman or a deliberate impostor. My friends and acquaintances in those days laughed at Tesla's claims, but something inside me would not permit me to laugh. Something inside me said, "Herein lies truth."

In 1897, the position for me changed. A dependable friend of mine – a well-known banker – told me of actual demonstrations of Tesla's electrical genius. My inner voice of confidence in the man began to take on the ring of truth. Tesla began to take on credence when such respected scientists as Albert Einstein began to give credit to his work.

Tesla had a dream that it would be possible to transmit electrical energy through the air without the use of wires. Some psychics declared that God would never permit such power to be released. Yet, my own intuitive convictions continued to tell me that Dr. Tesla was on the right track. In my personal position there was little that I could do about such matters, even though I most sincerely wished I could. I can, however, report succeeding events in Tesla's career.

The New York Times of 6 March, 1898, contained the following announcement under Tesla's own signature:

"After twenty-five years of labour and research I can affirm that I am well on the way to harnessing electricity and broadcasting it through space, and that other scientific technicians are well on their way to releasing the power locked within the atom."

Tesla's great discovery was that the harnessing of universal electrical power was through holding it in *rotation* instead of confinement. This was the *key* to mastering nature's tremendous forces. Such has been my inner intuitive conviction of the importance of Tesla's work all along. The greatest of scientific minds have equally held such intuitive convictions.

I will conclude this session on a wonderful note, in which I will quote from a private letter which I was privileged to read, in which Tesla tells of the mighty gifts of spirit which directed his life ...

"I have no power that is not communicated to me in the same way that any machine I may invent receives its power: through celestial radiation from the SOUL OF MATTER, the MIND FORCE OF THE CREATOR whose instrument I am. I know who is leading me and making all things work together for the good of all that IS."

While it is definitely a clairvoyant projection to a future yet to be, my spirit guides have told me that Tesla's dream will be realized in the unseen and given to the seen, when the time is right. Such power will be released on earth when mankind has reached such spiritual levels as to use such power constructively and not destructively.

....

177

CLINICAL REPORT

End of Session Twelve. Client aroused from deep trance pleasantly, of her own volition.

What can I say?

I briefly attempted to return to the subject of the repressed memories but my client would have none of it - another occasion perhaps, but only when she is ready.

Session Thirteen arranged.

Chapter Thirteen

MORE PSYCHIC CHILLS & THRILLS FOR ME IN 1898

Pre-session Interview. Carried out usual checks with client and had a far-ranging but general discussion of the content of the last session. My client was most surprised by the references to Tesla as she claimed to have no knowledge at all about the laws of electricity. Lots of talk about the world beyond the veil.

No mention at all by the client of the repressed memories so did not follow it up.

Regression session started in the usual way.

Session 13

I returned from BACK TO THE USA to my beloved England in 1898. My haunting adventures continued.

In the Spring of 1898, I made a trip to Ireland, and stayed a few days in Castle Rush. Some have said it is the most haunted castle in Ireland. It is one of the few old Irish castles still inhabited, very possibly inhabited by both the living and the dead.

At the time of my arrival, I was not feeling well at all. In fact, after taking one look at me, my kind hostess, Mrs. Kent who, with true Irish hospitality, thought more of her guest's well-being than of money in the purse, said to me, "Off to bed ye go, dahlin'. Ye need rest badly. We can tend to conventionalities later."

This had taken place after driving many miles and waiting drearily for a long time in a little inn in a small Irish town. The whole forty miles from that stuffy place to Castle Rush had been negotiated over very uncomfortable roads. I was most glad to fall in with my hospitable hostess's demand of, "Off to bed you go." I was soon tucked into my room. I now fully believe it was one of the haunted rooms in the castle but it looked very cheerful to me, and how good it felt to be resting on soft, downy pillows. It was enough to drive any thoughts of ghostly visitors from my head. I slept like a baby.

To tell the truth, although I knew the haunted reputation of Castle Rush as a hotel for ghosts – the investigation of which was a main purpose of my Irish adventures – at the moment my thoughts were miles away from ghosts. I had had a good night's sleep, and I was hungry. I called for breakfast.

Mrs. Kent obliged in a bounteous way.

Breakfast concluded, my Irish hostess called me to come quickly and see a curious sight through the window. It was raining "cats and dogs" outside. The rain was coming down in buckets. I could see nothing more than trees swaying, whipping wind and the drenching storm.

"Don't you see that girl over there?"

I looked again, and did see a girl just emerging from a clump of beeches, and carrying a small trunk upon her head.

"What a dismal day to choose for travelling," I said drily.

"Ah, that is Irish superstition!" rejoined my hostess. "That is my last kitchen maid you see, and she is so anxious to get away from this place that she is willing to walk seven miles in this downpour, sooner than wait a few hours here, when I could have arranged for a carriage to take her to the station."

"Is she mad?" was my natural comment.

"Oh no! Just desperately frightened. She has not been here even a week yet, and she is scared out of her wits. She is much too terrified to be coherent. All I can make out is that nothing on earth would induce her to spend another night at Rush. She says there are ghosts here. And whether she has really seen anything, or is only frightened by the stories of other servants, I do not know. Anyway, she certainly has the courage of her opinions, and is prepared to suffer for them! I would rather meet a dozen ghosts than carry that trunk on my head for seven miles in this pouring rain."

Then turning around casually to me, she remarked, "I suppose *you* have not seen or heard anything, Miss Bates, since you came? I hope not, for I am sure you are not strong enough yet for mundane visitors, let alone the other kind."

We were passing through the handsome circular hall at the time, and I said frankly, "Oh no! I don't think I should be allowed to see anything, even though I am a sensitive, when I do not feel wholly well."

Almost at the moment of saying these words something impelled me to place my hand upon a particular spot on the great stone wall by my side. "But there is something *here* I don't like," I said, tapping it – "something uncanny – but I don't know what it is."

Mrs. Kent made no remark, and I returned to my room. My entire stay at Castle Rush was most pleasant, and resulted in aiding my recovery. A few days later, I left to return to Oxford.

It was not until the following year that I was told by Mr. Stead that Mrs. Kent was over in England. She had been lunching with him and asking for me.

"She has given me a most graphic account of the way you "spotted" those skeletons hidden inside the wall at Castle Rush," he said.

I was completely puzzled by this remark. I had never spotted a single skeleton to my knowledge, either at Rush or anywhere else.

I told him so.

"She must have me mixed up with somebody else," was my final comment. "It is a kind of creepy place, in a way, and many of her guests might get a bit scared. But as for me she must have made a mistake."

"Well, I gave her your address, and she is writing to ask you to have tea with her at the club, so you can discuss it there," he said, and our conversation drifted into other channels.

Next afternoon, I met Mrs. Kent at her club, and I commented on the curious mistake she had made in telling our mutual friend, Mr. Stead, about the skeletons I had "spotted".

"But you *did* "spot" them," she said, laughing. "Don't you remember my asking you if you had noticed anything curious, or heard or seen anything during your stay at Rush? Do you not recall placing your hand on a particular spot in the circular hall and saying, "There is something uncanny here – something I don't like."?"

"Yes, I remember all that. But what of it? You never told me anything about skeletons."

"Of course not – your health was not up to discussing eerie things just then. All the same, your hand located the exact spot where my agent, only a week before your visit, told me two skeletons had been found sealed within the wall.

"It seems the former owner had found the skeletons hidden in the wall and he brought them out. However, instead of burying them, he bricked them up in the wall again. The story had got around about this, which was probably one of the reasons Castle Rush is regarded as being so excessively haunted."

She added, "All good psychics know that nothing disturbs a spirit more than disrespect for their funeral arrangements." I wasn't sure that I believed that, but anyway it was what she said, so I made no comment.

To return to Castle Rush:

Some years previously I had met, on an Orient steamer sailing from Ceylon to Naples, the Captain of the ship, who was the brother of the former owner of Rush. He was a hard-headed, practical sort of man. I appreciated the genial common sense of the man, and was grieved when I later heard of his death. Through him I came to know his family, and his sister-in-law was the one who wrote to me telling me that he had died under rather sad circumstances.

On the surface he seemed hard as nails, but underneath he must have been capable of deep affection. When I met him he had only been married for a few months. His wife died within two years of their marriage and, while visiting his brother at Castle Rush, he exclaimed: *"I shall not live a year after her departing, I know."* He was the last man in the world that I had ever met whom I would have expected to make such a declaration.

However ...

As his sister-in-law, in her letter to me, went on: "He was quite right in his prediction. *He died just three days within the year from the time of his wife's death."*

Beyond doubt, it was on account of my memory of him that I came to stay at Castle Rush on my visit to Ireland.

From Castle Rush I had planned on going to the south of Ireland to visit relations at Cork.

On the morning of my departure I was down in the drawing room, thinking about my being here at this old Irish castle. Nothing special seemed to have resulted from my visit. I did not even then know I had discovered two skeletons! Often in my life I have found some train of circumstances – a borrowed book, a stranger coming across my path, some unexpected visit - ordinary experiences that later turned into special experiences. I was really rather surprised to realize that I was leaving the "most haunted castle in Ireland" and that nothing had happened.

But in the very moment of saying this to myself, a curiously insistent impression came to me quite suddenly "out of the blue" as it were.

The impression was that the steamship captain, the brother of the former owner of Castle Rush, was urgently desirous to communicate something through me. As I was still feeling not fully recovered from my illness, I did not feel equal to taking any spirit message at the time. A long drive to the station and a weary railway trip lay before me, so I decided to do nothing until I was safely at my journey's end, in Cork with my relatives.

After a long, cold, wet journey, I arrived in a downpour (Ireland can be so wet at times. However, the trees and grass like it, which is why green is the traditional colour of the Irish). My kind cousin, who had come to meet me, was still patiently standing on the platform, but the conveyance he had engaged for me and my baggage had taken off.

This was truly a damp reception – it meant a thorough wetting for my cousin and me. Finally, another conveyance came by and he hailed it. Already seated were two people in addition to the driver, plus a heap of luggage including two bicycles. We squeezed in, but how we managed to make it is still a mystery to me. Suffice it to say, the miracle was performed, and we drove up the hill at an angle of about forty-five degrees into the bargain.

These surely were not ideal conditions for receiving automatic writing messages from the unseen world.

On arriving at my relatives' home, I gathered I did not look too well as, after having some hot broth, they insisted I go to bed. I soon forgot my troubles in a long, refreshing sleep.

When I awoke next morning I felt much better, and remembrance of the steamboat captain flashed into my mind. I found pencil and paper at once, in order to redeem my promise.

The message that came through positively affirmed that the castle was haunted – and that it would be well to tell the lady who now runs Rush to PRAY, PRAY, PRAY.

Now, this was not exactly the kind of message one would care to send to a rather recent acquaintance. When I had been staying at the Castle, two nice little girls had joined us at dinner. This comprised the family. I had been told another child was expected to arrive around Christmas-time (my visit was paid in September), but Mrs. Kent herself was convinced that this would be *another girl*, as she said rather sadly.

I sent the message to her at Castle Rush, with proper explanations.

I subsequently heard that Mrs. Kent was very interested in it, especially "PRAY - PRAY - PRAY," which apparently had great meaning to her.

I am glad to record that the child who later arrived was a boy, not a girl. He turned into quite an Irishman, and lords it over his elder sisters with his special brand of blarney.

That spirit message concluded my adventures regarding Castle Rush. Exactly how, why or what it was all about I frankly do not know. I do know though, that prayer can prove a most effective way of *laying* malicious spirits.

To this year belongs yet another strong psychic impression, left in a room which I occupied in the south of England following my return from Ireland.

It was a very comfortable room with nothing ghostly about it. However, it gave me an uncomfortable feeling that controversies had taken place there, and a lack of harmony hung about it in consequence.

I mentioned this rather tentatively to the master of the house – a very orthodox clergyman – and was told, "Oh dear no! Nothing of the kind. You are certainly mistaken."

But when I had the opportunity, I changed my room, and felt much more comfortable in consequence.

Several times I had noticed on the hall table letters which had come in addressed to another clergyman whose name I had not heard, and who was not staying in the house. Remarking about this to the housekeeper, she replied that the gentleman in question had lived in this house for several months, but that he had died a few weeks before my arrival. "He slept in the room you had when you first came. I was so glad when you changed your room."

"He was a clergyman, I see," I remarked as I glanced at the letters which had come in addressed to the reverend.

"Yes, he was ordained, but he had become a complete agnostic for some years. During the last few weeks of his life he had become very ill and had had to remain in bed. Reverend Dale, the owner of this house, was always going up there, and having long arguments and discussions with him. How much good was accomplished I really cannot say. All I know is that he died in that room."

As the housekeeper left, I pondered on this evidence of the truth of psychometry, in which a psychic atmosphere will cling to a room. No sensitive will question the fact, as it is a phenomenon clearly evident.

My friend, Mr. W.T. Stead of the Psychic Research Institute kindly allows me to mention another psychic incident connected with personal experiences of mine in the year 1898.

In the early part of that year, he lost his secretary – a loyal lady employee who had worked for him for many years. In an extreme fit of depression she committed suicide, by throwing herself out of a window in her flat. Two weeks previous to this sad occurrence, she had seen another resident in the same building throw herself out of a similar window. Mr. Stead has always feared that this acted as a suggestion upon her mind, following up one tragic example to her own tragic example. In other words, the first action led directly to the second action. However, her own accounting of the cause of her action differs somewhat from this impression, as you will notice when the case unfolds.

Mr. Stead was naturally sadly affected by the sudden death of Mrs. Morris, his secretary, and the circumstances attending it. While her body lay in the funeral parlour, he had some of her hair cut off, and sent portions of it to a dozen or more well-known clairvoyants, hoping to receive some solution to her mysterious impulse to end her life. They had arranged a secret sign between them, in the hope of obtaining objective proof of communication after death. Both parties were interested in psychic matters and agreed to honour no communications from the other side unless this secret sign was first given. As an investigating scientist, Mr. Stead fully appreciated the importance of such objective evidence.

Mrs. Besant, an intimate friend of Mr. Stead, was one of the clairvoyants consulted in the test. She had shown excellent perception on numerous occasions. She was confident of being able to discover details of the suicide, including revealing the secret sign.

Both she and the renowned Mr. Leadbeater were unsuccessful in the attempt.

In spite of the opportunity this test afforded for a clairvoyant to gain international publicity if successful, none of the dozen or more selected mediums were able to come up with the secret sign.

A few weeks later, following these unsuccessful attempts to obtain indisputable proof of genuine spirit communication from the other side, Mr. Stead and I were invited by an old friend in London to meet at her house for luncheon Miss Rowan Vincent, a non-professional sensitive.

I had never met this lady before. She was talking to several friends in her apartment when Mr. Stead and I entered. Completing her conversation with her other guests, Miss Rowan Vincent turned to me and said, very kindly, "Can I do anything for you now, Miss Bates? Shall I try to see anything for you?"

Something induced me, quite involuntarily, to say, "Do you ever get messages by automatic writing, Miss Vincent?"

"No, I have never done so, but I can try," she answered eagerly.

To myself, I sincerely reflected and hoped I had not sidetracked her into new channels away from her own special gifts. It was not that I had any special interest in automatic writing, but my impulse to request this form of mediumistic expression was entirely spontaneous. My interest was solely to see whether any from the *unseen world* could make themselves perceptible through this sensitive.

My suggestion of trying to communicate by way of automatic writing had taken firm root in Miss Rowan Vincent's mind, and she was determined to try the method.

She sat before a table on which was a pad of paper, and loosely held a pencil over it. I watched quietly and expectantly. Her hand holding the pencil began to move.

Soon she looked up, the writing having already begun.

"Do you know any William," she asked. "There seems to be some message from a William as far as I can make out."

Having a deceased Uncle of mine named William, I told her she might be correct, and that I would be glad to receive any message that came through.

A few moments passed, and then Miss Vincent said in a puzzled tone, "It is not *from* William – the message is *to* some William – I cannot understand it at all." She pushed the pad of paper rather impatiently towards me. Written upon it clearly but faintly was this message :

"DEAR WILLIAM – I want to explain to you how I came to fall out of that window.

"It was not my wish to do so. Someone or something pushed me from behind, yet there was no one else visible in the room other than myself at the time. ETHEL"

All this while, Mr. Stead had been standing quietly against the room's rear wall. His first name was William, I knew. He had not spoken, but his eyes gleamed with interest.

The signature was rather indistinct, so I asked Miss Vincent what she made of it. "It looks like Ethel to me," she said, "but it is not very clear. I will ask the spirit to write it again." A very bold and unmistakable signature was at once given.

I concealed my excitement, and said quietly to Miss Vincent, "I think I know from whom the message comes, and for whom it is intended, but to make sure it would be very satisfactory if the spirit could give through you a secret sign agreed upon by the sender and the recipient, and unknown to everyone else, including me.

"Well, I will try," said this non-professional medium. She had scarcely touched the pencil when it began to draw a circle. "There is no doubt about my having made a circle," she said, laughing. "Oh, now I am to put a cross into it," she added.

Mr. Stead dashed forward and scooped up the pad. With a broad smile on his face, he exclaimed, "That's it!"

Mr. Stead went on, his calm scientific demeanour coming to the fore, "Thank you, Ethel."

The three of us smiled.

That was it. A non-professional medium had done what the best in the business had failed to do.

I reflected to myself, "How very much are happenings in the *unseen* like happenings in the *seen*. In both realms, surprises do occur. How very much the Universe is like opening presents at Christmas-time."

....

CLINICAL REPORT

End of Session Thirteen. Again client roused herself by her own volition. Each session finds me doing less and less, and letting more and more just happen.

PERSONAL NOTATION TO MYSELF:

When I started this series of sessions with Sarah Channing in which she was regressed back into a lifetime when she was Katharine Bates ... I had no idea it was going to develop into such a ghost story.

Well, well, what next?

Session Fourteen arranged.

Chapter Fourteen

A RETURN TO INDIA

Pre-session Interview: Checked with the client about her experiences since the last session. Nothing important to report: everything seems to be under control. The client is now taking everything in her stride and we are very close to the point where she will no longer need me to guide her. Her knowledge of matters spiritual grows by the day, and we spent some time talking about some of her new discoveries.

At the appropriate moment Sarah moved over to the couch and promptly went into trance. Shortly afterwards she continued her story as Katharine.

Session 14

My second visit to India took place in the early months of 1903. I made it with my favourite girlfriend and travelling companion, Eleanor Greenleaf. I hadn't seen her for some time. She had been busy with her life, as I had with mine. But we had kept in touch and as soon as I wrote to her and said I was going to make a return visit to India, she was only too delighted to accompany me. So, here we were, halfway around the world together.

We approached India by way of Burma, as we were both anxious to see the world-acclaimed Shwe Dagon Temple. It is also called "The Golden Temple of Rangoon" and is a mecca for Buddhists from the four corners of the globe. We went there again and again, and wandered through its endless corridors.

Also:...

We spent several weeks upon the Irrawaddy River; wandered through beautiful, dusty Mandalay, explored Bhamo and marvelled over the exquisite vision of fairy-like beauty, painted anew for us each morning and evening, on this most glorious of waterways, and finally returned to Rangoon for a few days' rest before heading for Calcutta.

It was a lovely evening, just before our departure, when we went towards sunset to say farewell to the Shwe Dagon. At that hour it is to be seen at its best, for the rays of the setting sun light up the golden cupola into startling magnificence.

Having watched this glorious spectacle for some time the air grew chilly, compared with the intense heat of the day, and darkness came on swiftly as we turned to retrace our steps.

Down low in a dark alley, almost hidden behind the huge platform that supported the Shwe Dagon, was a grotesque, squat little temple. It was anything but beautiful, but there was a strange fascination about it. It sparked my curiosity, so Eleanor and I wended our way there and stood before it. A chilly draught seemed to proceed out of the dimly lit doorway. Taking a deep breath for courage, we entered it together.

I had no sooner passed beyond the doorway than I felt a most unpleasant influence. I wanted to run. I called to Eleanor, but she was staring in wide-eyed awe at a fantastic idol dominating the centre of the gloomy interior of the temple. Like the temple, it was squat and squatting.

In all my many years of travelling, I had never seen a god-creature like this one. It seemed to be made of gold and had four spindly legs and two spindly arms ending in large hands. It squatted upon a scarlet dais. It was so ugly it was almost beautiful, and it radiated power –

especially from the eyes. They were hypnotic. They almost seemed alive. It was those eyes that seemed to hold my companion in their grip. I tugged on her arm, but she did not move. There was something so malignant (no, that is too mild a word) – there was something so *evil* about the thing - that I started running out of the entrance, calling back to her, *"I can't stay in this place! I will wait for you at the top of the marble stairs."*

Now these steps, broken and dirty, and lined by small booths selling every imaginable kind of trinket, led via steep flights up and down from the huge platform to the ground.

I am, as a rule, rather a remarkably sure-footed person, and lanterns along the way threw ample light upon the steps, yet "something" from behind gave me a push, and I found myself falling to the bottom of the steps. I say *something* for there was nothing there. One moment I was groping my way down the steps, and the next moment I was flung through space. And in that moment, I had a flash of something I have never seen before in my life – I had a glimpse of another unseen world: it was a world ugly and dark and leering.

Naturally, through my occult studies, I had heard of daemons – creatures that hated mankind. Through my developing mediumistic perception I had seen the spirit world of my own kind. That was good. This world was definitely "ungood". The flash was gone, and I found myself, the breath knocked out of me, lying at the bottom of the steps, and Eleanor crying over me.

Fortunately, I was not seriously injured, although bruised enough to take several weeks to mend fully. With my friend's help, I got up and limped on my way.

I have had several falls in my life, but never one where there was absolutely no preliminary warning or a sense of slipping. The experience was exactly that of suddenly being *hurled down,* by some outside force, something out-of-body: there was certainly no person in-body anywhere near me that could have done it.

The short voyage from Rangoon to Calcutta was made pleasant by the kindness of a Rangoon friend, who came to see us off and offered to introduce me to a Burmese lady, very rich and devoted to Buddhism, who was on board with us.

"She is one of our most important native residents," my Rangoon friend explained before introducing her. "She is very interested in Buddhism and also Oriental mysticism. I think you will find you have mutual interests, from what you have told me of your investigations into spiritualism."

The lady was duly introduced to me and, thinking to open our conversation pleasantly, I remarked that I had heard she was interested in comparative religions and spirit phenomena.

Her reaction was the opposite from what I had been led to expect. She flatly stated, "I am very sceptical of the way in which your Western countries have pretended to understand our Eastern beliefs. I was personally acquainted with Dr. Grone, who gave a lecture on Buddhism in Colombo in which he said he was planning to become a Buddhist priest and, accordingly, had renounced returning to his wife and family.

The Burmese lady continued to expound the Grone mystery with some bitterness.

On their arrival in Colombo, she had arranged a room for him at the hotel, and had purchased some luxuries for him to make his new life at the monastery as pleasant as possible, as she fully respected the austere life he had chosen for himself.

However, when more than a week had passed and he gave no sign of moving in, she quietly intimated that it might be well to begin the new life without delay, and said she had contacted her brother, a priest himself, to meet Dr. Grone and present him to the authorities at the monastery. However, as he had made no effort to respond, she finally, in disgust, asked him to leave.

As a woman I could well understand her scepticism in regard to the sincerity of Westerners really wishing to learn The Way.

"Buddhism," she asserted, "is the way of the Master to advance mankind to Nirvana – the enlightenment of the human soul."

There is obviously some gulf of understanding between East and West in regard to such soul matters so, needless to say, I dropped any attempt to bridge that gap. So ... while on our trip, she, Eleanor and I enjoyed some social times. I let the spiritualism discussion drop into an abyss.

On arriving in Calcutta we parted company, and Eleanor and I went on to visit Simla. I found the atmosphere at Simla marvellous for psychic possibilities. However nothing of special significance occurred. Even Peshawar, with its glorious crown of snow-capped mountains, brought nothing in the way of psychic significance to me. Nonetheless my companion and I thoroughly enjoyed the second trek we were on, exploring "the land of magic". When we visited the Khyber Pass I fully expected to be haunted by the horrors of the past, but nothing of the kind came through. The beauty of the day when we visited this historic pass was only to be matched by its own extreme natural beauty, but no haunting memories hung there for me.

Our days spent in Northern India, at the base of the majestic Himalayas, might have brought some weird experiences, but outsiders, it seems, were seldom destined to extract magical phenomena from that enchanted land.

India often seems jealously to guard and keep her mysteries to herself.

As I look back on this, my second visit to India, it seems to me that Simla, even with its crowds of social butterflies (male and female) and dust and flies, and even the humid weather, still stands out to my mind as one of the most exquisite spots on Earth that the Creator created.

Not even the beauties of Kashmir have dimmed the memories of Simla for me. All beauty is sacred, and I guard jealously for myself, just as India guards her magic, my sacred memory of the place.

Although my return to India did not result in psychic incidents happening to me personally, one very personal happening did occur that made this trip one of the most memorable in my life. In was in Simla that I learned how to "go out of body" and take an astral journey. It is almost impossible to describe how fantastically remarkable it is to sense yourself floating in the air above your sleeping body and look down and see it there below you. It seems as though you are in two places at the same time. And astral travel is incomparable: you think of the place where you want to be and, with the thought, you are there!

And the "Silver Cord" is clearly visible in this psychic state, infinitely stretching from one body to the other.

CLINICAL REPORT

End of Session Fourteen. This is the fourteenth Prelife Hypnotic Regression Session with client, Sarah Channing. Client no longer requires hetero-hypnosis to enter the trance state and bring about recall of her previous lifetime experiences as Katharine Bates. She has already become a master of self-hypnosis. She relaxes, breathes deeply three times and instantly drops into trance. I need merely suggest, "Continue telling of your life experiences as Katharine." Immediate response. Clearly my client does not need me to teach her anything else about the process.

All she now needs is the self confidence to continue to explore for herself. Our last session together as agreed, Session Fifteen, arranged.

PERSONAL NOTATIONS TO MYSELF:

This session has proved one of the most significant of all, as two things occurred in it of great importance:

(1) As Katharine, Sarah had recall of intuitive glimpsing of a Parallel World – that of Daemons.

(2) As Katharine she, while in India on this second visit to that country, mastered the skills of going "out of body" and "astral travel".

PERSONAL NOTATIONS TO MYSELF:

In initial interviews with Sarah Channing, before our sessions commenced, she told of having, on occasion, experienced being "out of body" and mentally projecting to other places in space and time. It would seem that this talent, which she developed during the lifetime as Katharine, was carried over into her current lifetime as Sarah.

The "World of Daemons" can be considered *the dark side.* The "World of Angels" can be considered *the light side.* As Katharine, her soul automatically rejected the dark side and stayed with the light.

All force (i.e. energy) in the Universe is YIN and YANG (positive and negative), male and female, life and death, good and evil or, in religious expression, God and Devil. VIBRATION: this is the continuous movement from dark to light and/or light to dark. Without it the Universe would stand still. It is the perpetual vibration of creation. It is the VEIL between the seen and the unseen world. Through alteration in vibrational frequencies becomes possible SEEING THE UNSEEN. How wonderful it is to be a mystical-scientist, and not just a mystic or a scientist!

Chapter Fifteen

THE PORTRAIT IN GREBA HALL
& SPIRIT PHOTOGRAPHY

Pre-session Interview

Sarah Channing and I have worked together in this prelife regression experiment through fifteen sessions. In this last session, I have suggested she enjoy *anything* she would find interesting to tell about what happened during her lifetime as Katharine Bates. She has complete freedom in this last session to soar to wherever or whatever is her wish. Take it away, Katharine/Sarah ...

Session 15

I tell you truthfully, I have a special place in my heart for spirit photography. I am not speaking of fake spirit photographs, of which there are a host: double exposures, and that sort of thing. I am speaking of genuine spirit photography, when a manifesting spirit is indelibly captured on film. Genuine spirit photography provides an objective way of SEEING THE UNSEEN.

I will tell you some things about spirit photography, but first here are some interesting psychic phenomena centred around an old family portrait.

In the very heart of Warwickshire, there is a beautiful old half-timbered house, approached by an avenue of elms. The hall carries a history going back six hundred years.

The present squire is not only an old friend of my girlhood, but is connected with my family through marriage. He is the usual type of fox-hunting squire and country magistrate, who did good service during the South African War by raising a corps of yeomanry from the estate and going out with them to fight his country's battles, and he received a most hearty welcome from his family and his country on returning home all safe and sound. He is devoted to his splendid estate, and is one of the last men in the world, I know, to entertain fancies or superstitions about his house.

I must give this prelude by way of explanation before relating a psychic incident for which I find it difficult fully to account, except on the supposition that some real psychic sensitiveness exists under a hunting squire's "pink coat and top boots".

That half-timbered house of which I spoke is known as Greba Hall. I have known it since I was a child, and on its walls hang all the old family portraits. But there are so many of these pictures massed together that I could never distinguish one from the other, with the exception of a few immediate ancestors whom the squire brought to my attention.

Some years ago, I was staying with a lady who lived about three miles from Greba, and we drove over to the Hall to have tea with the Squire's wife, Mrs. Lyon. The lady whom I have mentioned had become interested in psychic matters since she had become acquainted with me, and I had discovered she possessed some psychometric ability.

Briefly, psychometry is the ability to pick up "impressions" and intuitions from the atmosphere surrounding any material object, such as a letter, a ring, an item of clothing and so forth. It seems that human beings are capable of impressing all material objects with the stamp of their *special* personalities. This seems to be especially true in the case of letters written and signed by a specific person.

The lady with whom I was then staying, Mrs. Fitzherbert, had tried receiving psychometric impressions from letters several times at my suggestion and had had good success. I mentioned this fact to Mrs. Lyon, and she suggested giving one of her letters to Mrs. Fitzherbert to be "psychometrized".

Mrs. Fitzherbert was sitting facing a door which led from the hall to an inner room, and over this door hung a good-sized portrait of an old gentleman. I had never particularly noticed it before, as it was hung rather high on the wall, and there had been no reason to call my attention to it.

Mrs. Fitzherbert glanced at the portrait, as she held the letter she was attempting to psychometrize. She gave a most excellent reading, and accurately described Mrs. Lyon's friend, both as to his character and rather unique conditions in life.

I was proud of her. She had done an excellent job. However, suddenly she complained of getting a severe headache. I knew she suffered from headaches on occasion, so I took her home at once.

As we drove in our carriage down the avenue of elms, she murmured to me in relief, "It's gone now. How thankful I am to get away from that old man! I knew he was telling me what to say about that letter, but afterwards he wanted to give me some message about himself. I could not understand it, and that is what brought on my headache."

Noticing my bewilderment as to what old man she meant, she explained, "You know, the old man in the portrait which hung over the door."

This was interesting, and showed some increased indication of her innate mediumistic powers developing. I suggested we had better try to find out what the old man wished to communicate, so we arranged to have a sitting for that purpose that evening after dinner but, as some unexpected guests dropped in that evening, we had to let this spirit questioning go until next morning.

By ourselves in the morning, Mrs. Fitzherbert and I sat down in the drawing room, armed with pencils and paper, to see if any automatic writing would develop. She suggested that possibly *I* should try to get the message, but I said "No" since she was the one who had received the impressions about the old man. She agreed, relaxed, dropped down into a quiet state and loosely held the pencil in her hand over the pad. It began to write, and the name of Richard Lyon was given, with the information that he had owned the Hall, and had passed over to the unseen world one hundred and thirty years previously. But when she tried to get further details, she was unable to grasp it, and passed the pencil and pad of paper over to me, to see what I could get.

Much to my surprise, he was able to write through my hand with great ease. He wrote, as the message came through, that he had been devoted to the estate, had lived to improve it in every way possible and, on account of the limitation of his life's purpose, there were many things he had failed to accomplish during his earthly lifetime. He then went on to say, in his writing, that he held fond remembrances of his beloved Greba Hall – it almost became his world.

"Could he be saying that he is "earth bound"?" suggested Mrs. Fitzherbert.

"Yes, that is the truth," was the eager response through my hand, "and it is sad to think that my own descendants are the ones who keep me imprisoned in this way. I am told that I could *progress*, as they call it here, and be much happier if I could forget Greba for a time. And it worries me to see things done so differently, and not be able to do anything myself for the old place. There is no happiness for me here. Do ask them to set me free," he continued rather pathetically.

"But they don't *want* to hold you down," I answered. "Tell me how they do it and what you want them to do?"

The old man's spirit then explained the position very sensibly. He admitted that his own deep affection for his old property and surroundings had produced a failure in his life to develop more purposeful objectives. This was one fault that must be overcome. Also he added, "That portrait of me hung in the hall causes a clinging to the past. It should be taken down. However, the picture may remain in England, provided it is not in any house owned by a *Lyon.*" (There were still several members of the family living in Warwickshire.) His spirit went on, "The portrait may be sent to London or elsewhere and kept by members of the Lyon family, provided they are not of direct descent, and did not live in my old county."

That ended the message.

We drove over to Greba that afternoon, taking the message with us. Mrs. Lyon was extremely interested. She not only endorsed what Richard Lyon had "told" us, and when he had lived, but also that he had done a great deal for the property. Her husband had often told her that and also that, on his death some one hundred and thirty years before, he had lain in state for three days in the centre of Greba Hall, and that his portrait had been hung in a place of honour over the doorway.

This was all useful information, so we all put our heads together as to *how* we could best help the spirit of this ancestor, and *how* best to comply with the old man's requests.

Mrs. Lyon remembered that several of the old portraits had recently been sent to a picture dealer in a neighbouring town to be cleaned, but this special picture had not been one of them.

Mrs. Lyon said, "I could possibly take it down and tell the men to store it for a time. But what would my husband say?"

I knew her husband, Squire Lyon, quite well. He was just the kind of stubborn, practical man who would say, "This spirit stuff is all nonsense. Of course we're not going to take the picture down. It looks good where it is."

I honestly hated to disturb the household, but I felt so strongly that something outside myself had inspired the message, with its definite instructions, that I told Mrs. Lyon it would be best to mention it to her husband.

She did so, and the refusal was as expected.

Well, I had done my best.

Several months passed, and the following spring I was once more in the neighbourhood, staying with some relations of mine, who were also related to the squire and his wife. There was happy news. I could hardly believe my ears, but I was told that the portrait had been taken out of Greba Hall and sent to London. It seemed that Mrs. Lyon kept mentioning it to her husband, and he finally agreed to take it down and remove it from the hall for a while.

"How did it all come about?" I asked.

I received the answer. "It seems that a few days after you left, the squire stood under the picture while waiting for tea in the hall. His wife heard him speak as he looked at the portrait of his respected ancestor. "Richard Lyon," he said, "Of course I know it's all nonsense, but would you really like me to take your picture down, and have you hung away from Greba Hall?" Naturally, there was no response from the picture, but something must have nudged him, for he gave orders to take it down and remove it elsewhere."

I have heard that everyone is happy now: the squire seems to have forgotten about the matter, and they tell me he is having a lot of fun doing up the estate.

I have frequently been asked how a picture could cause a spirit to remain on this side instead of moving on to its rightful state on the other side. I will explain as best I can.

The picture has no power of its own: it is simply a symbol of a lifelong devotion, to Greba Hall in this case. His was a lifetime of devotion to a special place and, at the same time, of being frustrated at not having done more *with* his lifetime than being devoted to the place. It represents a "push-pull" situation that causes lack of movement. The devotion to an old love causes a clinging to this side, while the desire to advance to more purposeful activities urges movement onward. The removal of the picture from Greba Hall to a new location breaks the cycle, thus allowing movement to take place.

Those to whom I have given this explanation seem to understand.

As to Richard Lyon on the other side, who can say? But I am sure the old gentleman is much happier now.

The spirit of the man represented in that old portrait brought in a great realization to me, which I repeated to myself: *"Do not become overly devoted to worldly things or they will deflect you from your life's path on this side and interfere with your entrance to the other."* And I recall the Master Jesus saying it so simply, in gist: "Seek ye first the things of the spirit if ye would enter the Kingdom of God."

Another psychic incident of interest that I recall occurred in the Autumn of 1905. I had been going through a period of stress, so I took some time off and went down to Eastbourne to get some peace. I arrived on the 11th of November, and the first few days brought rest.

Then a feeling of intense depression came over me. Why? I really did not know as, on the surface, things seemed to be going well enough. Still I felt depressed, and the depression increased.

Then, as suddenly as the depression had descended, it lifted. It was really a very profound experience, vivid and definite. As suddenly as they had enveloped me some weeks before, so did the heavy clouds now roll away, leaving me with a feeling of exhilaration. It was wonderful. It seemed almost as if I had escaped from a gloomy prison and was now able to walk in the sunshine outside. The curious thing about this complete reversal of my mood was that there seemed to be no special reason for it. Nothing had changed: my mood had just moved from black to white. In other words, the outer was the same, but the inner was different. Well, I cannot describe it better.

"But can't you account for it at all?" asked a friend who had been with me off and on during my depression period. He was delighted at the inexplicable change in my spirits.

Inanely, I found myself saying as a joke, "Well, it is the day after the shortest day."

We both laughed at my crazy comment. "What do you mean, "It is the day after the shortest day"?" he asked.

I shrugged my shoulders: "Honestly, I don't have a ghost of an idea." *Ghost of an idea:* I was getting closer to the truth than I realized.

To tell the truth, I had no special spiritual experience in connection with it, but I seemed to have experienced a happy feeling such as a child might have who had been lost and wandering in a forest, and then had finally found the path home.

Five days later, I read of the death of my esteemed friend, Dr. Arthur Hodgson, and received a letter from a colleague of his, giving some details of his last days. It mentioned that the Doctor had been very depressed regarding his work and other matters. Also, his health was slipping.

I began to understand the reason for my first depression and then subsequent elation. I had a soul-connection with this man. Through this rapport I felt his inner feelings. As he was dying in the *seen world* he was unhappy, as soon as he entered the *unseen world* he was joyous.

It was one of the most profound psychic experiences of a personal nature I have ever gone through. As an investigator of spiritualistic phenomena my curiosity led me to seek further details. I sent a wire to Mr. Stead asking what he knew of the matter. He replied that, like myself, his first intimation of anything wrong had been the report of the news of Dr. Hodgson's passing. I also wrote to Sir Oliver Lodge to get some facts. He kindly answered telling me that for some weeks prior to his death Dr. Hodgson had been very unhappy, as he had regarded his work only from the intellectual point-of-view. Sir Oliver sent me a copy of a note he had received from Dr. Hodgson a short while before he had died. It read:

"My work was intellectual – how could I regard it from any other point of view? That has nothing to do with the spiritual side of things. My spiritual life was latent, but it was sincere, as far as it went and, in this more favourable atmosphere, the buds are unfolding, and I am learning more and more of the love and wisdom which I always dimly saw and appreciated. It is the attitude of mind which is of paramount importance, and my attitude, though critical, was never obstructive, as you know."

"Change of attitude." There lies the key to the mastery of depression.

I wish to comment that this very personal experience of mine, sensing so strongly the emotional mood of one of my dearest friends, Dr. Arthur Hodgson, was directly connected with his mood as he approached his time of transition. It seems that, at that period, people often wish they had handled life in a different way than they had. I am certain from the way my feelings changed after he passed into the *unseen world* that his inner self recognized that he had truly lived a very productive life that time around.

This very intimate sharing of emotional moods between Dr. Hodgson and myself I can recognize as indicating the very close rapport I had with this special man, as I have already mentioned. As will be recalled when I told of my first meeting with him, there was an instant liking. The feeling was so instantaneous that it was a definite indication that I had known the soul, who was Dr. Hodgson, in some previous lifetime prior to my meeting with him in this current lifetime. The experience to me was far more than merely transfer of thought: *it was transfer of soul feeling.*

I should like to say a few words now on the subject of superstitions. We are *all* superstitious in various ways and upon different points. I may laugh at *your* superstition because it does not happen to appeal to me, but you may be quite sure you could find out that I have an "Achilles heel" too, in such regard.

The only difference between people is that some are honest about their superstitions and others are not.

I met a lady not long ago at a foreign dinner party who started our acquaintance by remarking that she was thankful she was not superstitious. While we were chatting at dinner, she absent-mindedly took a pinch of salt and tossed it over her right shoulder.

One of my own strongest spontaneous superstitions is my horror of breaking a mirror, with its supposed curse of seven years of bad luck to follow.

You may be assured that I am not so childish as to blame any bad luck I may have experienced upon breaking a mirror (and I have broken some during my lifetime) but, even so, I hold an instinctive horror of it that goes beyond my rational reasoning.

Again, I am quite aware that people may break a mirror, and it holds no more importance in their lives than that it means a replacement is required. I only maintain that, to *me*, it can portend *(and has portended)* some periods of distress.

Superstitions appear to be very personal to the individual.

When people say to me: "How can a sensible woman like yourself be so foolish as to think such things?" I can only truthfully answer that I would be very much *more* foolish if so many years of my life had passed without my noticing the sequence of events, but to *explain* the phenomenon is quite another matter.

I am not a scientist so I can offer no scientific or psychological explanation or evaluation of such occurrences. As a *sensitive*, however, it seems to me quite reasonable that, allowing that there is the possibility of influences coming to us from the other side, some sign – no matter how trivial – may be impressed upon us as a gentle warning to be prepared for some disaster. Many people sincerely believe they have a spirit guide or guardian angel who is with them during life, to help and protect them. What I am saying is directly related to this belief.

As we are discussing psychic incidents, here is an interesting one that I was directed towards by my distinguished friend, Oliver Wendell Holmes. As possibly you know, this man of brilliance had a sincere interest in psychic phenomena. It was at his suggestion, or at any rate with his approval, that I determined to pay a visit to a lady of whom he had spoken to me – Mrs. Arnold, a daughter-in-law of Sir Edwin Arnold. He informed me that she was a gifted clairvoyant.

I went to her house alone, so that she could not connect me with any mutual acquaintance. The subsequent interview was a remarkable one.

She told me of numerous personal happenings in my life that belonged entirely to my own private world of thoughts locked within my mind. She gave me a crystal ball to hold for a good five minutes, in order that it might become impregnated with my influence, then she took it from me and began making a series of statements without pausing for a moment or attempting to "fish", to use a popular term for trying surreptitiously to extract information from me.

These statements included my own life, studies, chief interests, the number and sex of my immediate family and also the attitude of various members towards myself. And, in each case, she was correct. She was an excellent clairvoyant.

Among her statements to me she said, "You are in great anxiety I see. It is about the illness of an elderly man. In fact, *two* people who are close to you are ill, I see, but I will tell you now of the one you wish to hear about especially."

She went on to describe not only my brother's surroundings and illness at the time, but also his permanent state of paralysis which was the result of his war injury, adding that he was now in the country, for she saw green trees all round him, and waving grass. As my brother's life for many years, since his forced retirement from military life, had been spent entirely in London and at the seaside, this was a good piece of objective evidence of her accuracy. As a matter of fact, he was spending a few weeks in a country cottage for the first time in his life.

The single point where she failed was as to the *time* of his passing onwards. She saw at once that the illness was one from which he could not permanently recover, and gave the approximate time very tentatively. "We cannot see times exactly," she said, "They only come in symbols. For instance, I now see falling leaves. It looks like an autumn scene, so I infer the time of his passing will be in the autumn of the year – perhaps October."

This, as I have said, was the only "mistake" of the whole reading. My brother passed to the Higher Life in September. Close perception.

When I saw his valet in town later, I asked him about the trees and he explained that there were in deed leaves all over the ground, which gave an autumnal look to every-thing.

Many people had noticed the same appearance in London and elsewhere. Fallen leaves came quite early in September of 1906.

The *second* friend lying dangerously ill was a puzzle to me at the time, but, within five days of my brother's transi-tion, I heard of the death of Judge Forbes, who was one of my most treasured friends, as Mrs. Arnold had truly observed. His illness was a very short one, but, on comparing notes with members of his family, I found he had taken to his bed three days *before* my visit to Mrs. Arnold, and was already seriously ill, although I had no knowledge of the fact for more than a week after my inter-view with her.

Now I will talk a little about spirit photography again, always a favourite subject of mine.

As my friend, Admiral Usborne Moore, observed in a letter to me: *"We are dealing with a great mystery here."* He is himself one of those who is working to solve the mystery.

It is a trait of human nature to give credence to our own achievements and be sceptical of those of others. This has very much been the case in relation to spirit photographs. We accept our "very own" psychic photographs as quite genuine and exclusive, but when a sufficient number of people are convinced by *their* personal experiences in this line of research, then people normally think that it is:
1. Impossible and absurd;
2. Possible but improbable;
3. Possible and not abnormal;

4. Possible, normal, *just what we all knew in the first place.*

Meanwhile, some of us have been experimenting with professional assistance, and in these cases the question is not, "Can such photographs be faked?": we all know that faking photographs is the easiest of all possible frauds. The real answer to the question must be determined by our recognition or non-recognition of the photographs produced.

As an example of this, if Mr. Boursnell or any other photographer can produce (as he has done) a spirit photograph of my old nurse, who died a quarter of a century ago, and who was never photographed in her life, then we must find some other suggestion than "fake photography" as a solution to the mystery. I have this photograph here before me at this very moment: there she sits as in life, with a little knitted shawl around her shoulders, and the head of a tiny child upon her lap. The eyes are closed and give a dead look to her face, yet the features are to me quite unmistakable, as no-one knew the dear old woman as well as I did.

To me, such stands as objective evidence as to the possibility of genuine spirit photography.

I flipped some pages and ran across, in my little album, another spirit photograph I love; it was of an old Oxford professor in whose home I had stayed many times.

Quite unexpectedly he appeared on one of Mr. Boursnell's plates last summer. The likeness cannot be denied. I compared the photograph with an engraving of a photograph taken earlier in his life. It appeared in a national magazine. With an artist friend (who had not known him) we went over the features one by one, and my friend said she noticed only one small difference, the exact length of the upper lip and this, she considered, could be amply accounted for by the lapse of time between the taking of the two pictures and the slight lengthening of the upper lip owing to loss of teeth. The professor passed away as an old man, which is how he looks in Mr. Boursnell's photograph; the picture engraved in the magazine represents him at least twenty years before his death.

But the most interesting point to me in this photograph is the appearance on his lap of a much-loved dog, a rather large fox terrier named "Bob". Bob was not only a very important person in the professor's household, but he was also fond of me, so it seemed quite natural that he should come with his master when the photograph was taken.

I remember arriving at the professor's home on one dark winter night to pay him a visit, and Bob's welcome to me was so enthusiastic he almost knocked me down.

I heard the professor say in a whisper to his wife, "Most touching thing I ever saw, that dog's greeting when Miss Bates arrives!"

Dear Bob! I am so glad he can still come and see me with his dearly loved master. Animal spirits in the unseen world? Why not? If we humans can be privileged to be there, why not our animal friends? The proof rests right here beside me.

Another photograph in my little album is that of a girlish face and figure, aged about sixteen I would say.

She first appeared on the photographic plate in the summer of 1905, but the face was so indistinct that I could not recognize it. A few months later the same figure appeared again, very clearly this time, and I could not help but exclaim, *"Why, of course, it's Lily Coleman."*

Now it is nearly thirty years since I met this charming child during my first visit to Egypt. She, her father (a distinguished physician) and her aunt were enjoying a holiday in Cairo, and I saw her often because she was the playmate of another girl – the child of a friend of mine at *Shepherd's Hotel.*

Lily was a delicate girl, with soft gentle blue eyes, and was always dressed in a simple, artistic fashion. A few months after our return to England I read in the papers of the death of this pretty child. I wrote a letter of condolence which was at once answered by the aunt, and since then I had seen nothing to remind me of Lily until this last year, when her photograph unexpectedly appeared upon the plate to again bring her to my attention. I am grateful to a wonderful Providence for allowing an influence as pure and beautiful as hers to be around me in my daily life.

And now let me conclude with these words:

Surely the aim of all psychic research should be to give us *scientific* proof of our trust in God, a spiritual foundation for the "HOPE THAT IS IN US ALL".

Spirit photographs and spirit manifestations amount to very little if we look upon them as an end in themselves, and not as the symbols of our continuing immortality.

I remember, years ago, having an absorbing conversation with Phillip Brooks, the then Bishop of Massachusetts, in which I asked him what he thought of modern theosophy, which was just then becoming a *cult* in his native town of Boston. There was a great deal of talk at the time about the new philosophy and the wonderful phenomena said to accompany it. Sir Edwin Arnold had written his "Light of Asia", and Oliver Wendell Holmes had welcomed it as something approaching a new revelation. People were talking about the historical Blavatsky teacups and hidden heirlooms found in Indian gardens, and some of us were wondering how soon we should learn to fly and what, goodness knows, would come next?

The Bishop's answer to my question: so genial, so characteristic, showing such divine common sense ... "It is not a question of *flying*," he said. "I should like to fly as much as anybody, and what a queer sort of bird I would appear!" He continued, "If you suddenly found you could fly, it would be *absorbing* on Monday, *intensely interesting* on Tuesday, *interesting* on Wednesday and *quite pleasant* on Thursday, but by the end of the week it would be getting normal, and you would go seeking some other new power. No, believe me, the real question is not flying, but WHERE YOU WOULD FLY AND WHAT YOU WOULD DO WHEN YOU GOT THERE."

This rather sums up the case in a nutshell, and to me seems only another way of saying: *"Don't forget the spiritual significance beneath the scientific symbol."*

And possibly I should add a philosophical thought which just popped into my mind: Let us all join hands in the interesting and absorbing work of trying to make our symbols as scientific as we can, by discovering the laws which govern them, as well as all the other things in our universe of Love and Law. Possibly we are here to learn that Love and Law are ONE. Possibly this combination is what we mean when we use the term GOD.

Well, this fairly well concludes my story of my lifetime as Katharine Bates. Thank you, Sarah, for being so patient, re-telling of my life in an age more spiritual than yours of advanced technology. What you have told through your recalled memories of me may help rekindle an interest in some almost forgotten arts of recognizing the "unseen world" which is continuously close beside us. And, if I may venture a prediction, the coming 21st Century, which will soon be upon you/me, will find mankind once again SEEING THE UNSEEN.

Thank you Sarah, but why should I thank myself – when you are me and I am you? It is all just a matter of illusory time, which in truth has no meaning at all in eternity.

However, before shutting off the memory banks and for completeness' sake, let's add an epilogue.

Epilogue:

The End Of A Lifetime

Time has marched by and, although I feel much as I did when in my thirties and was travelling about the world, when I look in the mirror and see the reflection of the body I now inhabit, I must admit it shows signs of wear. Elderly, I suppose, is what you would have to call it, and I recognize that physically now, I am no longer the girl I feel inside.

As I look back over my lifetime I can recognize what an interesting life it has been. Really, in some ways I have experienced twice what many people do, as I have had the opportunity to live in two worlds, while most people live in just one - two parallel worlds, existing side by side with just a wall of vibration separating them.

People have frequently asked me what has been the purpose of my investigating the psychic and the spiritual. The *purpose?* I would simply say: for my own enjoyment. My investigations have been much like a hobby to me. My hobby has been the human psyche. I suppose my hobby could have been collecting postage stamps, sea shells, fancy glassware and all manner of material things, but, in my case, the intangible has been of more interest than the tangible.

And possibly I should add this, which may comfort some who grieve over the apparent loss of someone they love: the truth is that there is no death at all, but just an ever-continuing of life, ever spiralling upwards. So know that loved ones wait to greet us, as the transition is made into the unseen world.

I left my body behind on 28 August 1914, and the most wonderful of all experiences it was for me. All my years as a sensitive were worth whatever travail such may have brought me at times. All was paid back a thousandfold by the opportunity this afforded me to make the transition (called death by those who do not know the actual truth of the matter) consciously. To be conscious of oneself going from the seen, passing through the veil, and into the UNSEEN is a glorious experience beyond any form of expression I can put into words.

My role as a psychic investigator has been completely unprofessional. I had the good fortune of being born into a wealthy family which gave me the freedom to do what I found interesting without having to scrounge for it. This freedom to pursue my hobby in any way I wanted has given me an opportunity to meet people of similar interests, make friends, enjoy some romance, have exciting adventures and investigate curious phenomena in diverse parts of the world:

PLUS

I was given a gift, which was like the icing on a cake, in increasing my enjoyment of what lies all about me, a gift of SEEING THE UNSEEN.

Our normal senses are so limited in detecting what really lies about us, and we sense so little. The unseen is even more remarkable than is that which is normally seen. What wonderful colours are there, what beautiful sounds. You can even understand animals' sounds and sometimes noisy chatter. Honestly, it is difficult to express in words what the gift of increased awareness has meant to me in the marvellousness of seeing the unseen.

Interplaying in two worlds is literally a doubling of consciousness. Really my life has been most fortunate, and I hope I have been able to convey some of that marvellousness to you in this reviewing of my life as Katharine Bates.

And, very possibly, the greatest bonus of all has been the realization that we are immortal, and that death is but an illusion that has no meaning in fact at all. In talking with people, so many whom I have met have such a fear of death. It is as though somehow they fear that when they die they will be extinguished just as a candle flame is snuffed out. Ha! Will they be fooled! For when they die they will find themselves still recognizing their personal individuality, and be even more alive than before ... for in a world of higher vibrations one is far less restricted than in the three dimensional forms of expression we are immediately familiar with. Here in the third dimension, we are truly limited. Think what it would be like to be living multi-dimensionally, in a world beyond time and space. Why, you could travel from Earth to Mars on just a whim of thought. Think of the perpetual fun of exploring the galaxies! And there is no need to be concerned with time, for you have eternity to get done what you want to get done. It is a world in which there is no need to waste your energy earning money, for there are far more interesting things to do than storing up banknotes. In such a world, money becomes just a meaningless jingle, jangle, jingle. And you come to recognize what you really are: a miniature of the universe, part of the CREATOR OF CREATIONS, part of ALL IN ALL.

And how nice it is to exist in a body free of aches and pains: a body in which ageing is impossible. Radiant well-being is yours there, always. And talk about love: if you think you know love in three dimensions, wait until you experience it in multiple-dimensions.

And yet, you know, it is strange but many so enjoy the ups and downs of life in the three-dimensional world that they insist on returning to it over and over again. Reincarnation. Actually such choice is a matter of where lies one's consciousness of what IS. For in the unseen world you can make a choice: of going upwards into higher realms of expanding consciousness, or of repeating the slower process afforded by third-dimensional existence. Which way you go is a matter of choice, for really there is no hurry. You have eternity. Every soul will ultimately head upward, but some prefer to move slowly, while others want to get there like a flash of light.

Well, enough of this telling of things you will eventually find out for yourself. It is probably best to let them come as surprises to your awareness, just like opening presents at Christmas time.

Last Clinical Observations

Having completed telling the story of her lifetime as Katharine Bates, subject stopped speaking in the cultured Oxford accent she had used in recounting these experiences, as an Englishwoman, and returned to consciousness as Sarah. As in all previous sessions she had total amnesia for all that had been told.

I make these notes for myself. There is no purpose particularly in reading them, unless from curiosity or interest. It is entirely up to you!

I must confess that Sarah Channing's telling of her lifetime as Katharine Bates, and then calmly stating as Katharine, "Thank you, Sarah, for being so patient, re-telling of my life in a more spiritual age than yours of advanced technology", makes me realize that the past knows the present, just as the present can come to know the past. Mind is so wonderful: there are occasions when it can even allow glimpses of the future. Remember the five diamonds the little bird brought Katharine?

Life is just a timeless continuum – each lifetime of experiences building upon the next in an ever-upward expression of higher and ever higher consciousness through ever-growing excellence in using the process we call mind.

PERSONAL

This last session terminated my personal research in exploring a series of previous life regression sessions with client Sarah Channing, born on 20th June 1957. Her lifetime as Katharine Bates concluded on 28 August 1914. This affords a time lapse of 43 years between her death as Katharine and rebirth as Sarah. Of that interim period (referred to in Tibetan lore as "the Bardo") I have no record.

This was the last session I ever had with the client. We had performed this experiencing of pastlife memory recall over a period of fifteen sessions. To my observation, it was evident that her inner mind considered that enough of her lifetime as Katharine Bates had been covered for her purposes at this time. I am certain the client will go on to develop her own psychic skills and will again visit her past life as Katharine. I have taught her all she needs to know to achieve this, and being in possession of a very active and enquiring mind I am sure she will.

These sessions with the client have brought home to me the real value of Previous Life Regression Hypnotherapy and Entity Removal Hypnotherapy. As a scientific clinician, I cannot precisely say what is my exact position of belief: that will require more investigation combined with objective proof, i.e. accuracy of places and dates mentioned, etc., as to whether such are fact or fantasy. I am inclined towards the former, as they present a testimony to our immortality.

SPECIAL CLINICAL OBSERVATIONS

Subject obtained more automatism as sessions progressed, but only aroused from hypnosis when each session had been completed although sometimes the decision was more hers than mine. There was no fatigue. Increasing ease (as a learning process, I would be inclined to say) for client to enter a subjective state of profound hypnosis (deep trance state of mind) with each session.

Questioning client at end of each session revealed amnesia in most instances, only on rare occasions were fleeting memories retained – much like a dream experience, remembering some at first, with a quick fading into subconsciousness.

I have recorded the entire fifteen sessions just as they were recited by the client. They are her property not mine, and so I asked her what she wanted me to do with her story. "Shall I write the story up?" I asked. She replied, "Do whatever you wish with it, but, if you write it, just stay with the truth, for honestly I do not know myself whether what came out of my subconscious memory is based on fact or fantasy. I suggest you tell the reader how it all came about, and leave it for them to have fun with reading it.

"Only please keep my real name out of it, as it is the kind of stuff that will interest the tabloids and cause me a lot of publicity. Out of the public eye, I live a very private life, and I do not want that sort of publicity. Also, it might make some of my close friends think I'm going nuts. Sometimes I think they think that already - just a little!"

IN CONCLUSION

As you have requested, here is your account, dear Sarah.

To me the most significance to be drawn from this research experiment is the factual evidence it presents that there is no death - death being but a change in energy fields in which the individual passes over to the other side, from the SEEN TO THE UNSEEN.

Ormond McGill
Palo Alto, USA
January, 1997

Postscript

Ormond sent me the first draft of this book in 1995 and asked for my views on publishing it. Whilst reading the manuscript many questions popped into my mind about Ormond's techniques, and also many other questions regarding his client Sarah Channing's experiences. Ormond was able to provide most of the answers but a number still remained and most of those could only be answered effectively by Sarah.

I was due to visit him in Palo Alto, California, later that year and asked him if it would be possible for him to arrange for me to meet Sarah. Initially Ormond seemed reluctant to allow me to see or even speak to Sarah on the phone, stating that he had not had contact with her since the last session in the previous year when he had obtained her permission to publish the material he had gathered about her life as Katharine. He also indicated that Sarah was a very private person and would be unlikely to want to talk to me about her experiences, so reluctantly I decided to let the matter drop but agreed to write a foreword to the book.

In October, my wife Glenys and I flew into San Francisco from New York, hired a car and drove down to Aptos, a small coastal resort a relatively short distance from Palo Alto. Our intention had been to spend a few days relaxing prior to meeting up with our good friend, Ormond. However, he had other ideas, called us up on the telephone and, knowing of our love of seafood, insisted on taking us for a meal at the famous restaurant located at the end of Capitola Wharf. He arrived accompanied by Chuck Mignosa, his long time assistant, and another close friend. Northern California was enjoying an Indian Summer and the temperatures were in the upper seventies. The meal turned out to be truly memorable, and we were treated to some of the finest specialties of the area. We had a lot to talk about, but towards the end of the meal Ormond leaned over and whispered, "I have a small surprise for you. Tomorrow afternoon you are coming with me to visit Sarah Channing". I was absolutely thrilled at the thought of being able to meet this lady at last. I was also a little mystified as he would not tell me where we were going except to say that it was quite a drive along the coast and he would call to pick us up from the hotel around midday.

When the meal was over we said our goodbyes and Glenys and I made our way back to our hotel. I then spent almost an hour racking my brain trying to remember every-thing that I had originally wished to ask Sarah. Eventually I felt content with the list of questions I came up with and hoped that the answers to them would tie up all the remaining loose ends of the story.

The following day Ormond arrived on his own, right on time. We agreed to take our hire car as Ormond had only recently undergone surgery to remove a cataract from his eye and he was still getting used to bright light. As I was now driving my first question was "where to?". "Monterey, but on the way we will stop off for some lunch in a bath tub which is located in a small place aptly called Pacific Grove." He chuckled. Ormond likes his little jokes, but I could not get my mind round this one. I guessed that if I was patient all would be revealed in due course.

A little over an hour later we arrived at the outskirts of Monterey and Ormond directed us to a car park outside a restaurant with the intriguing name of "The Old Bath House". Ormond announced that "a table was already reserved for us overlooking the sea." Walking into the restaurant was like entering a time warp as it was completely equipped and decorated as it would have been in Victorian times. Even the waiters and waitresses were dressed as they would have been a hundred years earlier.

We ordered a light lunch and, whilst we were waiting for the meal to be served, Ormond told us some more about Sarah. It rapidly became apparent why he had previously been reluctant to introduce me to her. Sarah was in fact a very well known public figure who went to great lengths to protect her privacy and steadfastly refused to discuss her private life in public. Sarah Channing was the name that she had used when she first approached Ormond and it was not until around his fourth session with her that Ormond realised who his client really was. This was familiar territory for Ormond who counts many famous figures amongst his past clients. Still Ormond did not reveal the true identity of Sarah.

Just after we had finished our meal a waitress came towards us bearing coffee. She placed four cups on the table and left. Almost immediately a lady in dark glasses slid quietly into the seat beside Ormond, gave him a hug, and introduced herself as Sarah Channing. As she removed her glasses, both Glenys and I were rendered speechless and reduced to doing what can only be described as excellent "goldfish" impressions, for sitting opposite us was one of Hollywood's best known actresses.

Sarah quickly put us at ease, apologised for the subterfuge and told us that since her regression with Ormond she had become a frequent visitor to the restaurant. She said she felt so very much at home there and had a wonderful feeling of the pace of life slowing down to a rate that she felt was just right for her the very instant she entered the place. So when she had had a very busy work schedule or just felt a little uptight this was the place she came to relax, returning to a pace that was more comfortable for her.

She went on to explain that the building had been built around 1890, and all the furniture and antiques were truly representative of the late Victorian or early Edwardian period. Many of the antiques had been imported from various parts of Europe and quite a few had come from England. On a previous visit to the restaurant she had been amazed to discover that, just by touching the various pieces of furniture, she was able to tell whether they had come from England, but could not give the origin of any of the other items.

Over coffee Sarah said that she would feel happier talking about her regression experiences in the privacy of her own home. This was just a short distance away, and she suggested that on the way there she would give us a short tour of Monterey and Pebble Beach and point out some of the interesting sights. So, with the permission of the owner of the restaurant, we left our car there and climbed aboard Sarah's Grand Cherokee Jeep.

The tour Sarah gave us was interesting in its own right as she pointed out the homes of a number of famous people including the mayor of Carmel, Clint Eastwood, and, a short distance away, the famous Monterey Lonesome Pine. There is no doubt that Monterey is a beautiful place sitting on the edge of the sea with incredible views and lots of beautiful trees. It is hardly surprising that it attracts people like Sarah to live there.

A little later we drove up a short driveway to some high gates which opened promptly on our approach. Beyond was a magnificent house set in stunningly beautiful grounds. The house itself was surrounded by tall trees but all around were an incredible display of flowering bushes and flower borders. We stopped at the front door of the house and got out of the Jeep. The front door of the house opened, and Sarah and ourselves were greeted by her housekeeper.

Sarah suggested that perhaps we could all benefit from a cool drink prior to talking about her experiences in exploring her past life as Katharine. Whilst the house-keeper went off to prepare our drinks, Sarah led us across the garden towards a gazebo which overlooked another separate terraced garden. Outside the gazebo were a number of chairs and loungers. We settled into these and Sarah said, "Well, where would you like me to begin?"

My first questions were about how and why she had sought out Ormond to do her past life regression and what her expectations had been. However, Sarah felt that, as the information I was gathering was to be part of this book, for completeness' sake it was necessary to go back to the beginning and her days as a teenager in High School. During that period Sarah had developed a really strong friendship with another girl in her class, named June. They had shared many things together during their process of maturing into womanhood and there had hardly been any intimate detail that they had not shared with one another. Sarah felt that this relationship had been really important to her during her High School years, as her parents were in the process of splitting up and she felt somewhat alienated from both of them. June had been through the same trauma some years previously and was able to empathise with Sarah, giving her the support that she so desperately craved.

The friendship had lasted down the years although they had both chosen different careers and had ended up living very different life styles in different parts of the U.S.A. However this had not stopped them communicating on a regular basis and meeting several times a year. June had married in her early twenties and had two children, a boy and a girl. Sarah had become godmother to both children and on many occasions had been told off by June for buying them too lavish presents, but she simply could not resist playing the role of "fairy godmother".

June's marriage was a very happy and successful one. Her husband Michael was successful in his chosen career as an accountant, had a good job and a nice house, and they had enough money to make life very comfortable. However, in late 1992 June became ill from what appeared to be a persistent respiratory infection following a bout of influenza. When this did not respond to antibiotics her doctor referred her to the local hospital, where her condition was diagnosed as cancer of both lungs. Sarah was not working at this time and immediately flew to be at her friend's bedside and also to help Michael look after the children. In a desperate attempt to find a cure for June, Sarah engaged the services of the best medical experts in the U.S.A., but to no avail, and June died in early 1993.

Towards the end of her life, June had several conversations with Sarah about the possibility of our existence continuing in some form after our death. Neither of them had strong religious backgrounds, but June knew that Sarah had always believed that there was something more to come after this life whilst she herself remained sceptical. A few days before June died, and when it was apparent that the end was near, she asked Sarah to consult a medium a little while after she passed on. June promised that if Sarah did this she would somehow make her presence felt from the other side through the medium.

This was obviously a very sad time for Sarah, and the memory of these events, although considerable time had now passed, still brought tears to her eyes. Sarah did all she could to help June's family recover from the trauma of losing a loving wife and mother, but shortly afterwards she had to return to California to start a new project. One day during a casual conversation with a fellow artist, mention was made of a clairvoyant/medium living in San Francisco who had assisted a close relative who had lost a loved one only a short time before. Sarah obtained the telephone number of the medium and vowed that she would call her as soon as she had completed her current work schedule.

Once her working commitments had been completed she returned home feeling totally exhausted and for a little while spent most of her time just sleeping and relaxing. As her energy slowly returned she began to feel an urgent need to contact the medium, so one afternoon she picked up the phone and called the number she had been given. She half expected to hear a recorded message or maybe a receptionist but instead she found herself talking directly to the medium. Sarah told her that she had been recommended by a friend of a friend to seek a reading and made an appointment under an assumed name to see her in a few days' time.

Sarah had long since learned to be wary about lowering her guard in circumstances like this so on the day of her appointment she took a number of precautions to conceal her identity. She is a master of disguise and is quite proud of being able to go more or less where she likes without being recognised whenever she wants to. Having prepared herself she exchanged her car for that of her housekeeper and then drove the hundred or so miles to keep her appointment.

She had only had one previous experience of engaging the services of what some people describe as a "sensitive", and this had been many years before. This had been at a time in her life when she had been very uncertain about her future and she had sought the services of an astrologer/clairvoyant in the desperate hope of obtaining some guidance. Now, many years later, she had very mixed feelings about what she had been told. So this time she had decided that she would provide the medium with only the minimum information about herself and that she would say she was there because she wished to know what the future had in store for her.

At the end of her journey she found the medium's house and parked the car in the driveway. As she walked up to the door it was opened by a lady in her middle years who introduced herself and invited her inside. She was taken through to a room decorated mainly with purple drapes and with silver and golden stars, moons and other astro-logical shapes hanging from the ceiling. In one corner was a large pyramid shape made from copper wire - this was hung with glittering crystals. Other large crystals of various colours were positioned round the room. In the centre of the room was a plain table covered with a simple black cloth. On the table was a crystal ball not much larger than a tennis ball and a pack of tarot cards. A chair was placed either side of the table.

Sarah was invited to sit on one of the chairs, and the lady then explained what services she could offer Sarah, but suggested that they start with a simple reading of the cards. Sarah found this interesting but of no particular relevance and very general in nature. At the end of the reading the medium asked Sarah to be patient for a few moments. She then placed both her hands palms down on the table and after a few moments started to rock backwards and forwards very gently. he then spoke in a low quiet voice. "I have someone here from the other side who wishes to speak to you. I believe his name is Henry. He says not to be disturbed for he knew you well when you were a child. He used to push you on the swing in your garden, and you used to squeal with laughter. When you were a little girl he bought you that great big teddy bear that you still have in your bedroom. He says he wished he had been able to stay on earth a little longer to maybe help you through the crisis of the family splitting up."

By this time Sarah was having goose pimples all over her arms and tears were rolling freely down her cheeks as she recognised the spirit as that of her grandfather. He had died suddenly from a heart attack when she was around twelve. She had loved him dearly and had felt a great loss for she had never had a chance to say a proper goodbye. Suddenly she blurted out, "I still love you Grampus. I wish you were with me now."

This did not seem to disturb the medium who continued, "Don't worry my dear, I never really left you. When you need me you can always find me standing just behind your right shoulder. But for now I have one last important message to give you. I have a young lady with me whom you knew as June. She wishes to speak with you but as she has only recently passed over and finds direct communication a little difficult, so I will convey her message for her. She says, "You were right Sarah, but it is taking a lot of getting used to. Please tell Michael I am fine and that he must get on with living his life without me. Give the kids a big hug from me. Thanks for keeping your promise. You and I will speak again shortly."."

With that the medium gave a deep sigh and sank forward resting her head on her hands. After a moment or two she sat upright in her chair and said, "That I believe, Sarah, is what you really came for." All Sarah could do was nod in agreement as she was rendered quite speech-less. "Just sit there for a few moments whilst I go and get us a refreshing drink, my dear," said the medium.

The medium slowly stood up asking Sarah what she would like to drink. On her return they sat drinking their drinks whilst the medium explained some things about the spirit world and why Sarah's friend had not communicated directly. She also told her that her grandfather appeared to be one of her guardian angels and that during the seance she had felt other spirits present as well. These had chosen not to communicate on this occasion.

Once they had finished their drinks the medium asked Sarah whether she was now feeling O.K. and would like to make another appointment. Sarah readily agreed and they fixed a date for the following week. As Sarah rose to leave she looked at her watch and to her surprise found that she had been in the medium's house for nearly one and a half hours, although it had seemed to her like only a few minutes.

Sarah returned for the next appointment and again her grandfather came through and gave her several reassuring messages but there were no more messages from June. Over the next six months or so Sarah visited the medium on five occasions. During these sessions her grandfather would have something to say and other spirits also put in appearances from time to time but none of these had any great meaning for her. During these visits to the medium Sarah learned more and more about life beyond death and the spirit world in general. Then one day, much to her surprise, after her grandfather had spoken he said June was there and wished to tell Sarah something. June first thanked Sarah for all the help she had given her children and Michael since she had passed over. She went on to say how glad she was that Sarah had taken an interest in the spirit world as this had played such a large part in her previous lifetime. Sarah then asked several questions but there was no reply from June until she came back with one final message and this was "keep searching for the truth, do not be frightened when you find it, as I will not be far away from you."

When the session ended, Sarah had many questions to put to the medium about past lives and how she could find out more about them. The medium said that the best person she knew to explore Sarah's own past lives was Ormond McGill and she gave Sarah his phone number. Shortly afterwards Sarah made contact with Ormond and the rest of the story is contained in this book. Sarah has not had any further sessions with the medium but does not rule out future sessions if she ever feels she needs them.

Having established Sarah's reason for seeking assistance from Ormond in the first instance I then concentrated on what had developed since her last session with him.

Sarah said that in simple terms her whole life had changed very dramatically. She was still continuing her career as an actress but had become more selective about the type of work she was prepared to undertake. This, she said, was perhaps not immediately obvious but she has always been very busy and her commitments stretched two years ahead. In the future she planned to do less work and have more time to herself. She also believed that she would be changing her role perhaps from actress to director or maybe producer if the right opportunity arose. She felt that she would not have been able to make such a decision had she not had the experiences with the medium and Ormond.

At a personal level she felt that for the first time in her life she knew who she was and what was really important to her. The words that she frequently used to describe how she felt about herself now were "integrated" and "at peace" as opposed to the past when she described herself as having felt "scattered and insecure".

Perhaps the most important discovery was that she now knew with absolute certainty that she was an immortal being and that, after this life ended, she expected to return in a new body at some future time. Another very important discovery had been her real purpose in this life. When I asked her what that was, her reply was "very similar to that of Katharine, which was to learn, teach and tell those who are interested about their true nature as immortal beings." Sarah referred me to her second session with Ormond where Katharine became aware of her mission in life.

She then posed a question for me. "How could my purpose be different from Katharine's? We are the same person. We just happen to be on earth in two different periods of time." I had to agree with her as this seemed completely logical given her story. I then asked how she was going to achieve her purpose in this life given her chosen career. She said that the first step had been co-operating in the production of this book but, unlike Shirley Maclean, she did not feel that it was appropriate for her to "go public" at this stage. When the time was right she would let the world know, when her spirit guides would no doubt point the way for her. For the moment she felt she had much to learn and was content to be getting on with this.

This led on to a number of follow-up questions concerning the connection between Katharine and herself. First I enquired whether she had continued to regress back to being Katharine using the technique Ormond had taught her. She said she had done so for a short time after the final session but now had no need. As she now felt integrated with her past life as Katharine she had at her disposal all the resources that Katharine had possessed in her lifetime. These included mediumship, clairvoyance and other spiritual gifts besides. At this time it was like rediscovering something wonderful from the past and she was still in the process of exploring this and getting to understand it better.

When I asked her if she had anyone helping her on this journey of rediscovery she replied that of course she had her friends on the other side, her Spirit Guides.

We then returned to the subject of integration. Sarah said that there were many obvious parallels between the two lives and suspected that Katharine could have been a great actress had she chosen the stage as her career. However there were aspects of Katharine's life and indeed her personality which were almost diametrically opposed to this life. A good example was their respective relationships with other people and in particular with men and sex. Katharine had gone through her life having only very superficial and non-sexual relationships with men. Her closest relationships had been with women, again non-sexual. In Sarah's case she had been married and divorced and had had other sexual partners. Sarah accepted that there was a huge gulf between the morality of Victorian times and today and perhaps that explained this. However, she was aware that her own sexual attitudes had been changing over the last year or so and she had no clear explanation for this. Initially she had felt it was mainly due to the shock and the grief at the loss of June, but pressure of work had also had a part to play. When we explored this more deeply it became apparent that she had made a very significant shift in her values and beliefs, which she now attributed to her growing spiritual awareness.

Many other values that Sarah had not previously doubted had also shifted and along the way she had also acquired some new ones. She described this as a process of evolution rather than revolution. She felt this was very appropriate, particularly as no great internal conflict seemed to have been involved, except one. Partially she felt this was due to her continuing contact with Grampus and occasional fleeting contact with June when she needed reassurance.

The one exception related to a really bad experience she had had soon after she had been "discovered" by Hollywood. This had involved her being raped by her co-star who had been almost twice her age and to whom she had not been the slightest bit attracted.

At the time they had been filming some really steamy scenes on location. It had been a very warm day and suddenly they had run into a whole series of technical problems with the filming equipment. Eventually the director in exasperation had called a break in filming for half an hour so that the technicians could get everything sorted out. She had gone back to her air-conditioned trailer to lie down and rest. She had been on her own and had shed all her clothes and had been wearing only a dressing gown when a knock had came on the door and there stood her co-star. He had asked her if he could have a few words about the script so she had invited him in. Once inside he had caught hold of her and tried to kiss her whilst she had resisted. He had then pulled off her dressing gown, wrestled her down on to the bed and raped her.

Sarah had been no stranger to sex but was deeply shocked and severely traumatized by what had happened to her. She was so badly affected that she was unable to continue filming for two weeks and was completely outraged when she discovered that she could do nothing about it as the whole thing had been covered up. Fortunately the director of the film showed a great deal of sympathy but she was forced to complete the remainder of the film with the rapist.

It is an enormous credit to Sarah as an actress that if you view this film there is no obvious sign of her performance being affected. However her experiences whilst on location had left very deep and lasting scars on her psyche. These had mainly manifested themselves in a powerful, burning hatred of the perpetrator of the crime. Over the years Sarah had lost no opportunity to attack him in any way that she could. At moments when he appeared to be receiving accolades from his peers, the critics or the press she would send him letters anonymously threatening to expose his evil deed.

The original attack and her hatred of her attacker had clearly affected her life in many ways down the years, some positively, as in her acting, but many negatively as, in some of her relationships with men.

During Session Eleven, Katharine had recounted her experiences in London in 1896 of the haunting of a Mr. Henry Halifax. On listening to the tape after the session, Sarah had drawn a number of conscious parallels with the servant girl involved. Sarah believed that the story had been true but that it had also contained a message to her in this life and that was to forgive her rapist. Initially she had tried to address the question by talking to Ormond about it but could not find the words that she needed in order to express herself adequately. It was clear to her that Ormond had also recognised she had encountered a problem. He had tried very gently to help her resolve it then and on other occasions but probably realised that she was not yet ready to face all the facts and make the necessary changes.

Shortly after her final session with Ormond she had "totalled" her car, when mysteriously a front tyre had blown out and she had had to be cut out of the wreckage. Fortunately no one else was involved and the airbag, seat belts and head restraint had all worked perfectly and all she suffered was minor shock and a few bruises to her legs. However whilst she was waiting to be freed from the car she found herself "going inside" and talking to her friend June. Much to her amazement June came through loud and clear telling her that the accident was just a reminder and that it was time to truly forgive, forget and get on with her life free from anger and resentment. All Sarah could say was, "Please show me how because I don't know how." Just at that moment the door was forced open and she was free.

When she arrived home some hours later feeling very tired and quite sorry for herself, she decided to have a soothing bath and go to bed although it was mid-afternoon. She quickly fell asleep and before long she began dreaming. She could not remember all the content of the dream but she could remember many spirits coming to her including Grampus, three other guardian angels and June all telling her what she had to do to forgive. The message was quite simple. First she had to forgive herself and she needed to do this because she had responded to evil by doing evil. She was told to go into trance and to find every occasion when she had done evil things to her aggressor and then to do the same for all the times that she had wished him evil. Finally she was to surround herself with pure white light and transmit love towards him. Then she had personally to go to her attacker to forgive him and to ask for his forgiveness.

A few days later she went into trance and carried out the first part of the task. When she came out of trance she felt as though a great weight had lifted from her shoulders. That night she asked her agent to obtain the phone number of the actor concerned. The following day the agent called her back and a week later she found herself entering the actor's house. She felt no fear or apprehension; she had the feeling of almost walking on air as she walked into his home. A maid announced her arrival to her employer who was sitting in a high-backed leather chair looking for all the world like a character from a nineteen thirties Fred Astaire and Ginger Rogers film. She noticed that he looked pale and drawn and a whole lot older than when she had last seen him the previous year at one of the awards ceremonies. He ushered her to a seat opposite him and offered her some refreshment.

Sarah explained that she had contacted him again because what had happened all those years ago still bothered her, and she wished now to meet him face to face to put the matter to rest once and for all. "Well my dear," he said, "if you had come to see me in a year's time you might have left it too late. My doctors tell me that I haven't got much longer on this earth. I've got Aids and my time is running out real fast now. I guess I've made my last film. In fact there's a whole bunch of things that I won't be doing any more, including loving. My only hope now is they find a cure real fast for this goddamned disease."

Sarah was completely shocked by what she heard and for a moment was completely lost for words. All she could say was, "That's real sad."

"Oh, don't be sad," he said with real meaning. "I've had a great life. After all sixty-six or sixty-seven's not a bad age to go. It's a hell of a lot nearer three score years and ten than twenty-two and I nearly didn't get to make twenty-two. I very nearly had my ass shot off in Korea when I was twenty-one; two bullets missed my butt by less than a couple of inches. So every year since twenty-one's been a sort of bonus, if you know what I mean. More to the point, I don't have too many regrets either, but I do have a couple, and one concerns you. Do you mind if I talk about this first because it's clear that it still bugs you and is the reason you are here?" Sarah was still finding the right words hard to come by and just nodded in reply.

"Well, I guess I have never really figured out what happened that day when you got so goddamned mad at me for doing what I thought you really wanted all those years ago." Sarah suddenly found her voice and blurted out, "I never expected you to rape me."

"That's the point," he replied. "I never thought I had! I really thought you had the hots for me because of the way you had played the previous scene. You were comin' on so strong I couldn't believe it was all acting. It was all a terrible mistake, but I never got the chance to explain or say sorry till now. You really must believe me. I have always felt sorry that it happened but I am even more sorry that it hurt you in the way that it did. Can you forgive me after all these years?"

242

"Of course." she replied. "But the reason that I am here is to say sorry to you for all the hurt that I have caused you. Can you forgive me?"

"Too right, and by the way, I know who I got this disease from and I've forgiven her. You don't have to worry. It was a long time after we made that film together," he said, slowly getting up from his chair. "Now just to finish off putting the whole world to rights would you make an old, sick man happy by giving me a long but ever so gentle hug. I just feel like I need a little warmth and love in my life right now."

Sarah got up, put her arms around him and burst into tears and a moment later she was aware of his tears running down the back of her neck. At last they had resolved a misunderstanding that had caused both of them a lot of pain down the years. They stood like this for several moments. Then he said, "Thank you, my dear. I'm feeling quite tired after all this talk and must go and rest for a while. If you happen to be passing this way, do come in and see me. You will always be welcome."

Sarah left the house feeling a mixture of relief and sadness but above all with a feeling of inner peace. A couple of weeks later whilst reading a book just prior to going to bed she had what many would perceive to be a strange experience. For a brief, fleeting moment she clearly felt he was there with her in the room. She stood up and instantly felt just as though he was embracing her in exactly the same way as when they had last parted. After a few moments the sensation slowly faded away. The following morning it was announced on the television that he had died the previous evening. She knew that he had come to say farewell to her on his journey out of this life.

This experience had a profound effect upon Sarah. Now she felt confident that she had been empowered to use her latent skills handed down from her previous life as Katharine. She was developing these daily, and to prove her point she gave Glenys and myself a reading of what life had in store for us in the next year or so. Some of the things she told us were very specific such as that we would move our offices to larger premises, although at that time we had no plans to do so. Recently we moved our offices! Many of the other predictions she made have similarly come true.

On our return to the United Kingdom Glenys took on the task of trying to find documentary evidence of the existence of Katharine Bates. Despite a considerable amount of detective work and research on her part little progress was made other than the discovery of vague mentions of Katharine in a number of late Victorian journals. Close to the point when the book was due to go to the printers Glenys discovered that there was definite proof of Katharine's existence. This came in the discovery that Katharine had been the daughter of the Reverend John Ellison Bates, rector of Christ Church, Dover, Kent. There is also evidence to suggest that Katharine contributed articles and papers for various psychic magazines in the late nineteenth century. Among these was an address written by her entitled *The Psychic Realm - Wanted a Constitution*. She had been invited to write the paper for a convention in America in 1898 to celebrate the Jubilee of Modern Spiritualism.

Since the discovery of this information, Sarah has said that, although she was aware that Katharine had a penchant for writing, she always believed that it had taken the form of a diary. She is also absolutely certain that she has never read anything that could have been attributed to Katharine Bates, and her knowledge of Victorian or Edwardian history was very scant.

As Sarah is not yet prepared to reveal her true identity, our research must, for the time being, stop here. On a therapeutic level clearly Sarah has benefited considerably from her experiences. How much of this benefit is directly attributable to past-life regression alone and how much is attributable to Ormond's brilliant covert counselling is difficult to assess. However there is no doubt that the regression clearly has played a major part. She herself has made that quite clear both in the answers she gave and by her own assertions that she now feels psychologically stronger and more balanced. How matters will progress from here, who can say? Much will be dependant upon the choices that Sarah herself makes on her continuing journey through life.

Thank you most sincerely, Sarah, for the help that you gave me which enables me to produce this Postscript. My hope is that it will add a completely new dimension to the life that you related as Katharine. I really believe that this should be the starting point of a book about you, Sarah. Or, if not a book, how about a film?

Martin Roberts Ph.D.
Wales
February, 1997

Appendix

Appendix

TRANSCENDENTAL HYPNOTISM
INDUCTION

This is the first publication of my Transcendental Hypnotic Induction. As this technique provides the subject with an insight into his or her divine nature and immortality of BEING, I am including it as an appendix to this book in order to provide a further means of extending research into this important phase of hypnotic phenomena.

Often a person will consider his body as himself, and that is not the truth. Man is not just a body at his roots. He is an individual CONSCIOUSNESS and, through his mind, his consciousness becomes known. A body is but an instrument used to conduct our affairs in the physical world. Transcendental Hypnotic Induction brings about this realization.

Have the subject take a seat in a comfortable chair, place his feet flat on the floor and rest his hands in his lap, so they will not touch. The light in the room should come from behind the subject directed towards yourself, as the hypnotist. Give these suggestions:

"As you sit quietly in the chair, relax every muscle of your body. Just let yourself go. As you do this, direct your attention to my eyes; look deeply into my eyes, and keep your complete attention fixed upon my eyes, until I tell you to close your eyes.

"As you stare deeply into my eyes, notice how your perception of my eyes begins to change. It begins to seem that, instead of focusing upon my eyes, the point of focusing moves through my eyes - to the other side of my eyes - to a point far beyond my eyes. You will find that you are no longer looking at my eyes, but that you are looking through my eyes into myself. It is as though my eyes have become windows through which you look directly into the space which is inside myself. You are becoming aware that you are looking through the windows of my eyes out into the vastness of space – in which the stars of the heavens pulsate and shine.

"Let your entire body completely relax now, and send your BEING through the windows of my eyes and project your BEING into that vast space which spreads before you.

"As you look deeply in this manner while relaxing your body completely, your eyes become so heavy and completely relaxed that you can no longer hold them open, and your eyes close. So close your eyes. (Eyes close). It feels so good to close your eyes now, and relax completely all over. Your eyes are closed now and are so relaxed that you cannot open them no matter how hard you try. Try as you wish, but you cannot open your eyes. So try no longer, just relax into the vast space which you see spreading before yourself even now that your eyes are closed.

"Now ...

"You feel yourself sinking down into this vast space which spreads before you infinitely. But your eyes are closed, so you are no longer looking into my space ... the space you now witness is your own space. Deeper and deeper you sink down into this vast space of yourself. Every breath you take sends you down deeper and deeper, down into this vast space of yourself which is independent of the physical world. Your breaths are deepening, and every breath you take sends you down deeper and deeper into this vast space ... far, far down beyond even a vestige of consciousness of the physical world.

"Drift. Drift. Drift. You find yourself drifting in space. A mind free of its body in this space ... drifting down ever deeper and deeper into space.

"Now ask yourself some questions as you drift down into this vast space. Are you the one who is called by a certain name in the physical world? Are you the person who lives at a certain address? Are you the person who possesses a certain bank account and holds a certain position in the world? Experience how you feel right now in this vast space in which you now experience yourself ... this vast space which is beyond the physical world. And all the things that you thought you were suddenly come to have no meaning at all ... for you are now a free mind drifting in free space. You are none of the things that you thought you were, and yet you are still YOU.

"As a free mind, you are drifting down deeper and deeper into this vast space. And to where do you experience yourself drifting? You are drifting down to the very centre of this vast space; you are drifting down to the very centre of yourself.

"You are drifting down, down to your SELF ... going deeper and deeper into the vast space of yourself. You see your SELF before yourself, and you ask a question, 'How can this be ... for I am here in space drifting down to myself?' And suddenly you realize what you really are - you are the consciousness of your SELF, and you appreciate and recognize this fact with great joy in at last knowing – in full awareness – what you really are. You are an individual consciousness, and you appreciate and recognize this fact with great joy in at last becoming fully aware of what you really are – that the SELF you see before you, in this vast space, is the real YOU, while the you which you had previously thought was yourself is but the mind which that SELF uses. This insight comes upon you like a bursting of stars ... and suddenly you feel utter blissfulness, utter peacefulness, utter happiness ... and you find yourself dropping down directly to that CENTRE OF YOUR BEING, which is your SELF.

"You go on down, down into your SELF, and you merge as one BEING. In doing this, you experience complete rest, for now you are home. Now you know what you really are and what you are meant to be. Now you know what you really are: YOU are the mind of this SELF - the consciousness of this SELF - through which YOU manifest.

"Now ...

"Even this realization begins to melt and fade away as you melt into yourself ... and you experience no longer a separation of yourself as being mind on the one hand and as being SELF on the other ... for your mind and your SELF have become one, as pure consciousness. Each is part of the other which combine as consciousness. NOW YOU KNOW BEINGNESS. And along with this experiencing of your BEINGNESS you also experience your relationship of oneness expanding to include oneness with all that is the Universe. Suddenly you KNOW THAT YOU ARE PART OF THE TOTALITY: that a part of that totality is YOU ... that YOU ARE THE TOTALITY ... YOU ARE ONE WITH THE INFINITE.

"This experiencing of SELF that you now know completely changes your relationship to the physical world in which you live at this moment, in the here and now, and that, of course, includes your body. It gives you a control over your body that you never before imagined you possessed – for now that you as mind and you as self work together as a team in complete unity, the SELF takes over control of the mind, as it manifests in the physical world. And the mind now under control of the SELF makes you a master of your mind – a MASTERMIND which can bring perfection to your body, as is your wish.

"With this control which you now have, you can make of yourself whatever you desire. You can heal your body, you can keep your body in perfect health, you can reform its habits, you can make your body perform to a perfection beyond your wildest dreams. You can master ALL that is about yourself, and achieve whatever you desire to achieve. You have discovered yourself and, fusing mind with SELF, you have established SELF as the controller of mind, and you become THE MASTER SELF.

"Now ...

"You have discovered who you really are, and you can cause all concerns and worries to vanish and disappear forever, as is your wish. You are now in complete control of yourself, and you have the power to make of yourself exactly what you wish to be. From this time on, you will control yourself always from your CENTRE OF BEING ... and you will make of yourself the perfection which it is your right to be.

"This which you now know as truth, from having personally experienced this truth, will stay with you always. Every breath you take into your physical body automatically reinforces this truth, and causes it to become your realization. You know yourself as being in perfect control of your health and well-being.

"I bring you back now to the here and now on a joyous returning to the physical world with this blissful KNOWING burning within you like an everlasting flame."

References:

TEXTS RELATED TO PASTLIFE HYPNOTHERAPY

Bolduc, Henry L. *The Journey Within: Past Life Regression and Channeling*
Independence: Adventures Into Time, 1988

Bolduc, Henry L. *Self-Hypnosis: Creating Your Own Destiny*
Independence: Adventures Into Time, 1992

Bolduc, Henry L. *Life Patterns: Soul Lessons & Forgiveness*
Independence: Adventures Into Time, 1995

Cheek, D.B. & LeCron, L.M. *Clinical Hypnotherapy*
New York: Grune & Stratton, 1968.

Cheek, D.B. Maladjustment Patterns Apparently Related To Imprinting At Birth
American Journal of Clinical Hypnosis, 1975, 18.

Cheek, D.B. Short-Term Hypnotherapy For Frigidity Using Exploration Of Early Life Attitudes
American Journal of Clinical Hypnosis, 1976, 19.

Cheek D.B. Techniques For Eliciting Information Concerning Fetal Experiences
Paper presented at the meeting of the Society For Clinical And Experimental Hypnosis, Los Angeles, California, 1977.

Dethlefsen, T. *Voices from Other Lives*.
New York: M. Evans and Company, 1977.

Erickson, M. & Rossi, E. *Experiencing Hypnosis: Therapeutic Approaches to Altered States*

New York, Irvington 1981

Fiore, E. *You Have Been Here Before*.
New York: Coward, McCann & Geoghegan, 1978.

Imich, A. *Incredible Tales of the Paranormal*.
New York: Bramble Books, 1995.

Kelsey, D. & Grant, J. *Many Lifetimes*.
London: Corgi, 1976.

Kubler-Ross, E. *Death: The Final Stage Of Growth*.
Englewood Cliffs, New Jersey: Prentice-Hall, 1975.

Kubler-Ross, E. Foreword. In R.A. Moody (Ed.) *Life After Life*.
Covington, Georgia: Mockingbird Books, 1975.

LeCron, L.M. *Techniques Of Hypnotherapy*.
New York: Julian Press, 1961.

Leonardi, D. *The Reincarnation Of John Wilkes Booth*.
Old Greenwich, Connecticut: Devin-Adair Company, 1975.

Moody, R.A. (Ed.) *Life After Life*.
Covington, Georgia: Mockingbird Books, 1975.

Moody, R.A. *Reflections On Life After Life*.
New York: Bantam, 1977.

Netherton, M. & Shiffrin, N. *Past Lives Therapy*.
New York: Morrow, 1978.

Ritchie, G. *Return From Tomorrow*.
Waco, Texas: Chosen Books, 1978.

Rossi, E. L., & Cheek, D.B. *Mind Body Therapy: Methods Of Ideodynamic Healing in Hypnosis*
New York: W.W. Norton, 1988

Rossi, E.L. & Rossi K.L.   *The Symptom Path To Enlightenment: The New Dynamics of Self-Organization in Hypnotherapy: An Advanced Manual For Beginners*
   Pacific   Palisades,   California   Palisades   Gateway Publishing 1996

Stevenson, I.   *Twenty Cases Suggestive Of Reincarnation.* 2nd Ed.
   Charlottesville, Virginia: University Press, 1974.

Stevenson, I.   <u>Some Questions Related To Cases Of The Reincarnation Type</u>.
   Journal of American Society of Psychic Research, 1974, 68.

Stevenson, I. The Evidence Of Man's Survival After Death.
   J. Nerv. Ment. Dis., 1977, 165.

Van Husen, J.E.   <u>Development Of Fears And Phobias In The Fetus Following An Attempted Abortion: A Case Study</u>.
   Paper presented at the meeting of the Society for Clinical and Experimental Hypnosis,   Los Angeles, California, 1977.

Wambach, H.S.   *Reliving Past Lives: The Evidence Under Hypnosis.*
   New York: Harper & Row, 1978.

Wambach, H.S. *Life Before Life.*
   New York: Bantam Press (197?, now out of print)

Watkins, H.H.   <u>The Development Of Ego States In The Fetus Following An Attempted Abortion: A Case Study</u>.
   Paper presented at the meeting of the Society for Clinical and Experimental Hypnosis, Los Angeles, California, 1977.